# Yoga From
# the Inside Out

# Yoga From the Inside Out

## MAKING PEACE WITH YOUR BODY
## THROUGH YOGA

*Christina Sell*

Foreword by John Friend,
Founder of Anusara Yoga

HOHM PRESS
Prescott, Arizona

Cover design: Kim Johansen
Interior design: Book Works, San Diego, California

**Library of Congress Cataloging-in-Publication Data**

Sell, Christina, 1969–
Yoga from the inside out: Making peace with your body
through yoga / by Christina Sell
p. cm.
Includes bibliographical references and index.
ISBN 1-890772-32-1 (pbk.: alk. paper)
1. Yoga. 2. Body Image. 3. Yoga—Therapeutic use.
I. Title.
RA781.7.s4346 2003
613.7'046—dc21
2003000537

HOHM PRESS
P.O. Box 2501
Prescott, AZ 86302
800-381-2700
http://www.hohmpress.com

This book was printed in the U.S.A. on acid-free paper using soy ink.

07 06 05 04 03     5 4 3 2 1

*To Lee Lozowick,*
*the best yoga teacher there is.*

# Acknowledgments

To adequately acknowledge all of the love and support that have contributed to the writing of this book is an impossible task. Be that as it may, here goes. I offer my gratitude and a very special thanks to:

Lee Lozowick, for, well, Everything.

John Friend, for believing in me and for helping me to be strong and soft. You rock.

Desiree Rumbaugh, for showing me how much fun it is to practice yoga. You are a great teacher and a great friend.

Manouso Manos, for pointing the way.

My husband, Kelly, for being my best friend. I love you. Thank you for being a great photographer and for helping all of the models feel beautiful. Thank you for knowing when I had to write and understanding when I couldnít play. Thank you for loving me.

My sangha-mates, for Refuge.

The Anusara Yoga Kula, for the absolutely incredible ways that you lift me up out of my self-centered suffering and for the laughter.

My yoga students, for inspiring me to live up to what I am teaching. Thanks for sharing the journey with me.

Everyone who shared their story with me. Whether or not your interview is technically "in print," I used every conversation I have had on the subject to write this book. Thank you for your willingness to be vulnerable and to reveal yourselves so thoughtfully.

The models who posed for the pictures, for your commitment to the project and for loving yourselves. Your beauty is blinding.

Allison and Howard Kravetz for your personal and professional support. Your friendship is a blessing.

My editor and mentor, Regina Sara Ryan, for all you continue to teach me about communication. I think you are the coolest.

# Contents

# Foreword

BY JOHN FRIEND, FOUNDER OF ANUSARA YOGA

The glory of the Arizona rising sun just above the horizon shone directly into the entryway of the yoga studio with such flooding brightness that I couldn't make out any details of the person who crossed through the threshold into the room. Yet it was clear that the darkened form walked through the blinding blaze with the compact power and lightness of a splendid tiger. As a young woman stepped out of the direct sunlight and into the center of the yoga room she welcomed me with a radiant smile and sparkling eyes. Her lustrous skin seemed to vibrate with pure potential energy condensed in a short, stocky, athletic body with a strong countenance that reminded me of '84 gold-medal gymnast Mary Lou Retton. I offered back a big, open-mouth smile as I approached to shake her hand and find out her name. Silently I thanked Divine Spirit for allowing me to encounter this amazing embodiment of the Supreme on that dazzling February morning.

Her name was Christina Sell and all I saw before me was the tinkling delight of Spirit incarnated in a vibrantly fit woman who could easily do a standing back flip right there in front of me if she wanted to! It was not until a few minutes later, as my Anusara Yoga Intensive in Scottsdale got underway, that I saw the deep sadness in her eyes, and the fearful warrior mentality in her solid muscular body. Within the first couple of poses it was clear to me that Christina was arguably the strongest and most in-shape student in the class, yet when I offered her a compliment on the beauty of her poses she glanced at me sideways with utter disdain. How does it happen that a beautiful, super fit, talented yogini thinks so little of herself?

One explanation for poor self-esteem is provided by the viewpoint of tantra, which serves as the philosophical basis of Anusara Yoga. In the tantric view everything in the world, including our ephemeral bodies, thoughts and feelings, is seen as a manifestation of a singular, eternal Spirit, whose essence includes pure Goodness and Beauty. However, in the never-ending process of creation this truth becomes concealed and forgotten. Instead of seeing ourselves as ever-lovingly held in the grand embrace of Supreme Spirit, we perceive ourselves as essentially alone and separate from others. Yet, our innate spiritual interconnection creates an unconscious burning desire to belong and feel liked and appreciated by others. So, we attempt to make ourselves attractive to others based on society's superficial definitions of beauty, success, and power. Advertising agencies and the media inherently define what the most popular look and image is, and we then often use this definition as a measuring standard for ourselves. Many times this arbitrary standard sparks self-hatred and a war with our body when we feel that we are far from what it takes to be "attractive" or "popular."

At the time, I wasn't sure of the reasons, but it was clear by Christina's forceful attitude in her poses that she had a war going on with her body. I also sensed that she expected me to join with her against her body, to criticize her poses and tell her about all the imperfections that I observed. However, to Christina's surprise, instead of taking a narrow view of her poses, I took in the whole form first, without looking for postural details. With delight I simply admired the magnificence of Spirit shining through the artistic beauty of every part of her yoga poses. Instead of disapprovingly noting all her postural misalignments, I stood quietly, smiling, in front of her for a few seconds, and then summarized my assessment of her yoga pose with one soft word, "sweet." It was a perfect moment —there was nothing more for me to say; and nothing more for Christina to strive for in her pose. In that moment an offering of peace was made and a ceasefire began in a war that had been waging internally for many years. Coming up out of her pose, eyes filled with tears, Christina seemed to relinquish the muscular armor that she had been laboriously wearing for a long time. Her jutting granite jaw slackened and her body visibly softened like a baby's. For a few minutes the transformation that was beginning inside Christina seemed to be heralded outwardly by the sunlight becoming noticeably brighter throughout the room.

Now, three years later, Christina moves on and off her yoga mat with an unbounded freedom and ease, and with laughter in her eyes. Tremendous energy and focus still vibrate in every pose for her, but now instead of trying to forcefully make her body fit an image-standard established by some outside authority, Christina playfully aligns her poses in ways that enhance her innate beauty. She adjusts her postural alignment not to fix something wrong with her pose, but in order to allow Spirit to more fully flourish in her unique form of the Universal. It is truly by the power of Grace that her war with her body is over, and she now feels the wonder of Spirit coursing through her body with every breath.

May the Grace and wisdom that fills every page of this book help you to shine your own divine beauty in your life from the Inside Out!

# *Introduction*

*Before we can find peace among nations, we have to find peace inside that small nation which is our own being.*
—B.K.S. Iyengar

This book is about yoga and body image. More specifically, this book is about the journey through the issues of addiction, self-love and spiritual practice. One year into my study of Anusara Yoga, a style of hatha yoga that integrates "Universal Principles of Alignment," the art of inner body awareness and the celebration of the heart, I wrote an essay, "about what I was learning in and through my yoga practice.

I shared a copy of this essay with John Friend, the founder of Anusara Yoga. Several weeks later he read the essay aloud during an intensive workshop. I felt many emotions as the words of my life story were anonymously read aloud to seventy people. I felt the pain I had lived with my whole life—the pain of hating my body, of doubting my essential worthiness to such a degree that my body became a battlefield in my desperate attempts to prove myself worthy

# Anusara Yoga as a Peace Offering

I am six; my best friend's brother violates my body. I am nine; I am so sore from gymnastics camp that a hot bath is necessary every morning to get my body moving again. I am ten; the calluses on my hands have ripped from the uneven parallel bars. I am encouraged to continue training until my hands bleed. I am eleven; I am in a cast due to tendinitis from over training. I am sixteen; I am binging and purging many times every day. I am seventeen; I am drinking heavily and using drugs. I am eighteen; I am acting out sexually. I am twenty; due to compulsive overeating, my five-foot-one-inch body now weighs over one-hundred-fifty pounds. I am twenty-six; I am competing in triathlons. I am twenty-nine; I am training for a bodybuilding show with hard workouts and strict dieting.

I am thirty; I hear John Friend tell us that "every pose is an offering." A revolution begins to take place inside of me.

Perhaps I am jumping ahead of myself. I had done yoga before this particular workshop. I knew a decent amount about technical alignment and about the form and shapes of the poses. I was reasonably strong and flexible. I was familiar with yoga philosophy and had done a fair share of chanting. But after five days at the intensive with John, I realized that I had never done yoga from the inside out. I had

of love and to numb myself to the fear that I was fundamentally flawed. I felt compassion for myself for how much I had struggled. I felt hopeful and grateful for what I was learning and for the new relationship I was developing with my body.

Most importantly, I began to feel a layer of shame being lifted from me. As John read, people nodded, cried, and re-

been approaching my yoga the same way I had learned to approach everything—with force, criticism, and by ignoring my pain. Quite clearly, I saw, I had been perpetuating a war against my body so profound that my heart broke open at the tragedy of it. Like any war, there were casualties—after all, one can't wage war on the body without such violence affecting the mind, the spirit, and the emotions.

And so I cried. For five days at the intensive I cried. For three days after the intensive, I cried. I cry now as I write, but for different reasons, a year later. I cry now because I am grateful. I cry now because I am learning to practice differently. I practice setting my intention that my yoga mat is sacred space. I practice more restorative poses and I no longer lift weights, train for long races, starve or over-feed my body. I practice telling myself what I am doing well. I practice accepting my yoga and myself as I am, indulging in less criticism and less faultfinding. I practice softening more and hardening less. And I laugh more. I practice asking God that my yoga be an offering of peace to my body. Every time my hands come to *Anjali mudra*,[‡] I can offer peace to my body and honor it as the temple it is. When something hurts, I practice looking into it, rather than ignoring my pain. In these ways, I know I am honoring my body and myself. I am making peace.

[‡] Anjali mudra: a hand position, placing palms together, fingers extended, pointed upward, in front of the heart—a gesture of prayer and offering.

ceived my story with compassion, understanding and empathy. The effect of such a response was that I felt blessed, understood, and transformed by the power of the group's acceptance. I was able to see the many different people in the room all relating to some aspect of being at war with the body and the self. I knew I was not alone.

Returning home from the intensive, I had many conversations with my yoga students and friends about their issues with self-acceptance, body image, compulsive exercising and food related struggles. Some people shared with me that they were in the throes of their own personal war. Others describe surfacing from the depths of their process with insight and reason to celebrate. I began to realize that I had something I could offer people who were dealing with the issues of body image, self-love and spiritual awakening. I envisioned a book that would honestly describe the ongoing struggles that many people have with their bodies and their self-esteem, and how the practice of yoga helps them to manage these challenges.

I dreamed of a book that would honor and celebrate those who attempt to end a war with themselves. Hopefully the book would expand our perception of beauty and offer us a chance to glimpse a greater possibility and purpose in and through the practice of hatha yoga.

I have written the book that I have needed to read. In so doing, I have realized the age-old adage that "You teach best what you most need to learn." Be that as it may, this book is my offering of peace—to myself and perhaps to someone else who is ready to practice the yoga of self-love. In Sanskrit, the word *abhyasa* means "tireless practice with devotion over a long period of time." Surrendering to the demand of abhyasa is the real message of this book. Making peace with the body is a practice, not an event. The practice is a journey through which we confront our fears and our conditioning, and receive the opportunity to glimpse the greatness of our true nature.

# CHAPTER ONE

# *War and Peace*

I was six when my best friend's brother sexually abused me. Over a period of several months he and his friends involved me and his sister in sexual fondling, games of a sexual nature, and watching pornographic films. I never said no nor did I ever tell anyone about what was happening. I understood these events to be a secret and I experienced the confusion of feeling physical pleasure concurrent with the shame and fear typical of children who are sexually abused. Over time I kept the abuse a secret, even from myself, as these memories were hidden from me until my early adulthood.

I was the youngest child in a family that placed a tremendous emphasis on being thin and on watching one's weight. I was a physically small child. My older sister, Anne-Marie was round and soft in her physique. Our parents put Anne-Marie on a diet when she was nine. My interpretation of these dynamics was that thin was good, fat was bad. I assumed I would be more lovable if I stayed thin.

Being intelligent, logical and highly verbal, I was successful academically. Being small and physically coordinated, I was naturally suited for gymnastics, and also participated in dance, soccer, softball, and violin and piano lessons. During pre-adolescence, competing in gymnastics at the state level, I first learned to push past my body's limits, to ignore my pain and to pursue perfection through the physical body. (In retrospect, I have no idea why we were pushed so hard as young gymnasts. We were already past the age where Olympic competition was possible and clearly this was an extra curricular activity, nothing else.) During this time, on the physical level, I dealt with various over-training injuries, ripped calluses on my hands, constantly sore muscles, sprains, bruises, and aches. I even broke my front tooth in practice. Emotionally, I learned to pursue perfect scores. I grew accustomed to competing with other girls for the coach's attention and for the

*Ustrasana.* Camel pose.

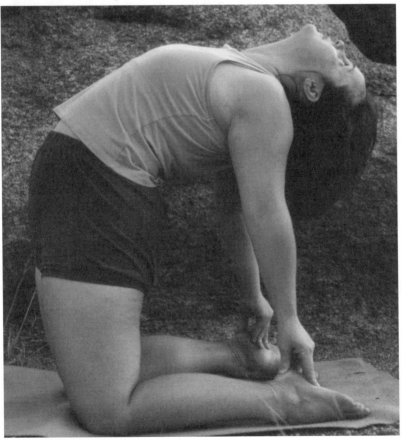

judge's approval. I learned that thin and cute was better than plain and heavy. I learned how to be perky, to smile and to act happy regardless of how I felt. I became accustomed to being the center of attention with a judge constantly deducting points for each mistake that I made.

As puberty arrived, I lost interest in the demands of gymnastics training and switched my efforts to socializing, cheerleading, and popularity at school. And though the external scenarios changed, I had by this time internalized the judges, the competition and the perfectionism of my gymnastics training. I no longer needed outside forces to push me and to demand that I ignore my pain.

At sixteen, and after a series of painful events including the break up of my first sexual relationship, I faced an existential crisis. I felt depressed, hopeless, unlovable, and scared of growing up. I developed a stomach ulcer that required a special diet. I began losing weight. My slender body attracted attention from the boys at school. My pain and depression increased and I began to purge the food I was eating. I soon began to binge and purge daily. The patterns of my bulimia included binging on large amounts of food, self-induced vomiting, over exercising, the use of laxatives, diuretics, alcohol and drugs of all kinds, stealing and sexual promiscuity throughout high school and the year following my graduation. I was obsessed with food and compulsive in my eating patterns. Although I was desperate to stop the binging and purging, I was unable to manage my behavior and I felt totally out of control.

My late adolescence and early adulthood marked the beginning of a process of recovery. At eighteen and, seeking help for my depression and bulimia, I enrolled in a sixteen-month residential therapeutic program for young adults. I worked intensely on my issues of low self-esteem. I stopped purging, abstained from alcohol, drugs and sex and I began the process of growing up. I was introduced to 12-Step Recovery and to the functional concept of a "higher power." I also began teaching aerobics and running long distances. I managed my eating excesses primarily through exercise. This period of my life was full of growth, change and improved health. However, the mental obsession with food, calories and the criticism of my body remained intact. I still binged and I often ate beyond the point of feeling full. I gained forty-five pounds.

Throughout my early and mid-twenties the acuity of my bulimic patterns lessened. Years of abstinence from purging followed years of struggle with binging weight gain, weight loss; periods of excessive exercise contrasted with periods of moderation. I was introduced to yoga when I was twenty-two and began an intermittent practice over the next five years. The years where I primarily practiced yoga for exercise were years in which my bulimia was less acute.

By my late twenties I was training for and competing in mid-distance triathlons. At twenty-nine, I had re-entered the fitness "industry" world. I was teaching aerobics and indoor cycling, and preparing for a bodybuilding show. Not surprisingly, I was developing over training symptoms. I was obsessed with my physique. Once again I was engaged in an addictive relationship with exercise. Occasionally I binged and purged.

At this time my body was an ideal specimen—the epitome of the goals of the fitness industry. I had approximately 11 percent body fat, my muscles were sculpted and defined, and I was tan from long hours spent in the tanning booth. Everywhere I went I got compliments on how I looked. My exterior looked as close to perfect as it ever had. However, I was tired, constantly hungry, irritable, and unfocused. My muscles ached, the plantar fascia on my feet were so tight it was painful for me to walk. I was obsessed with my body, terrified of gaining weight, and my husband was telling me I was not as much fun as I used to be.

Attending a yoga workshop with my main yoga teacher at the time, a senior instructor in the Iyengar tradition of hatha yoga, he adjusted me in a pose. All of a sudden I was flooded with emotions and grief. I began to cry and my teacher asked me if it was physical pain. I said no. In fact, I was aware that there was not even a story line connected to the emotions at all. My body was simply releasing stored feelings. I continued to stay in the pose, following my breath and taking instruction from my teacher. Before leaving the workshop that evening, my teacher told me to not be afraid as I would go through changes. He said, "You know, your challenge has never been strength or your willingness to work hard. You are good at those things. What you need to do now is surrender."

## The Surrender

By the age of thirty I was no longer bodybuilding. Along with teaching indoor cycling, I had returned to yoga with more dedication and was teaching classes locally. I had begun to realize that the cost of my perfect physique was one that I could not afford to pay. While I hoped that one day I would be able to accept looking more average, mentally, my obsession was still quite strong. Emotionally I was missing the approval that my physique once brought me. I gained fifteen pounds.

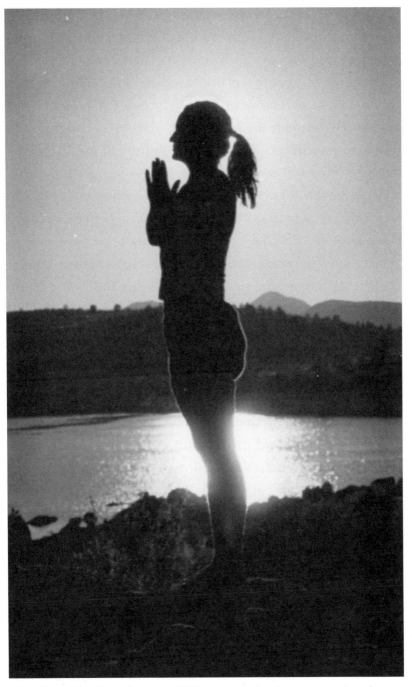

*Anjali mudra in tadasana.* Offering mudra in mountain pose.

One evening my husband and I were in the coffee shop where he worked and as he cleaned up the counter I began eating some of the pastries. Not paying attention to the amount I was eating, I began to feel overly full and I thought to myself, "No matter, I can throw it up later." The familiar internal struggle ensued between the bulimic self and the recovering self. From past experience I knew that if I purged I would feel immediate relief followed by shame, remorse, and disappointment in myself. I knew I would have to work myself out of a very familiar hole of self-loathing. On this particular night I knew, stronger than I ever had before, that I did not want to go through that process one more time. I made a cry for help!

During this period in my life I was just beginning to approach a particular spiritual teacher, studying his books and learning about the lineage he represented. My teacher's spiritual master was an Indian saint named Yogi Ramsuratkumar —a beggar who lived on the streets of southern India. This night, caught in the internal debate of whether or not to purge, I remembered that the old beggar had said that if anyone needed help and invoked his name that he would be there. My cry for help was to him—I begged for Yogi Ramsuratkumar's intervention with as much strength as I could muster—and the compulsion to purge that evening was lifted. Yet, by the time I got home with my husband, I had already forgotten about the miracle that had just occurred.

The following day, while I was teaching an indoor cycling class, I looked up and saw a woman who was preparing for a bodybuilding show. She was pedaling furiously. I noticed how developed her muscles were becoming. I thought sadly that I would no longer have this look since I had stopped lifting weights and I was making an effort to eat more and to exercise less. Suddenly my mind switched. I thought to myself that I didn't even really *like* the way she looked. Her physique, right before my eyes, began to appear overly developed and man-like. I saw hardness not only in her physical body but in her emotional body as well—a grip of fear and an unnecessary intensity drove her, reminding me of the pain that motivated me through such grueling workouts. She looked bizarre and distorted to me. I thought to myself, aren't women supposed to be softer, rounder? Suddenly I was aware that the grace I had asked for the previous night was continuing its work on me. My ideal was being changed right before my eyes. I felt the presence of Yogi Ramsuratkumar. I knew in that moment that the saint was altering my preferences for the appearance of the female body, and especially for my own body.

A miraculous event was occurring from the inside out. Never before had my standard for my body been one of round curves and softer features. I had periods of differing weight; I had experienced varying degrees of destructive acting out; I had long stretches of healthy eating and moderate exercise. But my ideal for my body had never been different than that of the cultural norm. Later that day, as I wrote to my spiritual teacher about what happened during the class, I realized I could not turn my back on the profound implications of this new way of seeing.

## *The Peace Offering*

One month after the remarkable event of a changed perception, I attended a five-day Anusara Yoga Intensive with John Friend. He asked us to set an intention for the week. I thought of my spiritual teacher, Lee Lozowick, and how

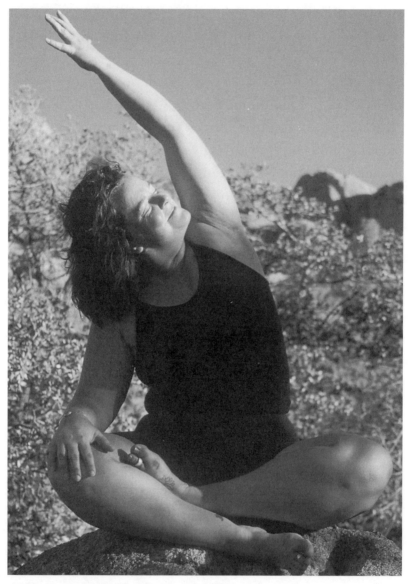

*Ardha padmasana variation.* Half lotus variation.

I wanted to become closer to him. John talked about making every pose an offering. He talked about draping our outer body over the radiance of our heart. He instructed us in how to create psychological balance for ourselves by practicing with the proper intention. He peppered his discourse with directions about physical alignment but he was primarily focused on something he called our *bhavana*—a Sanskrit word that addresses the feeling state of the pose and of the practitioner. He asked us to consider what our pose might communicate or express emotionally.

Prior to this workshop I had studied yoga primarily with teachers who emphasized precise alignment. John's approach was different from my previous training. He was telling people they were great and commenting on the strengths of people's efforts, not their shortcomings. I was shocked. My rational mind was critical—he was neglecting to tell people they were making mistakes! However, emotionally, I was softening. Tidal waves of grief welled up inside me. Since the teacher wasn't yelling, I could see more clearly how *I* was the one who was always yelling at me, and *I* was the person who was constantly criticizing my own efforts.

I had the added gift of an injury during the Intensive. I had hurt my shoulder a year earlier in another yoga workshop and I had lingering pain in the joint. John kept explaining that the key to yoga therapy was to put the body into correct alignment and to keep it properly aligned in each pose. When I applied this technique, the pain went away. However, in order to find correct alignment in each pose, I had to slow down and pay very close attention to my pain. Obviously, being slow and paying attention to my pain were new practices for me. The very practice of paying attention to my pain, coupled with John's ongoing insistence that every pose was an offering, and that the body was an expression of the Divine, began to shatter the protective armor I had around my heart.

I saw that every time I had ignored my pain I had basically ignored myself. I saw that I had been trained throughout my life to perpetuate a war against my body that had also pushed me to ignore my very being. The realization of how deeply I had hurt myself and how I had not only abused my body but also neglected my spirit was profoundly sad to me. I grieved for the little girl I was and all I had experienced, as well as for the woman I was and all I had missed because of my obsession with perfection and the harshness with which I had treated my body. I knew that I had to find a new way to practice yoga. I knew I could not go home and behave in the usual way.

One night John asked us to write about what offering we could make with our practice. I realized that if I practiced in a way that ignored my pain with harsh and critical internal dialogue, I would be perpetuating the same war that I had known my entire life. I realized that if I could learn to slow down, to pay attention to alignment, to honor my pain and respect my limits, then I could make my yoga into an offering of peace.

## Keeping the Peace— Ongoing Negotiations

Upon my return from the yoga intensive I realized that the ongoing peace negotiations for me meant entering more deeply into spiritual life. I formally became Lee Lozowick's student and began learning about how to live in relationship to a living guru. Through my interactions with Lee and his students I became aware that many of the principles necessary to practice hatha yoga as a peace offering were integral to his path as well. Central to his teaching is a radical reliance on

## Rachel's Story

The history of my relationship with my body has been a road (or maybe even a roller coaster) of destruction and abuse. My mind has formed many judgments about my body over the years, often pertaining to society's expectations that I look a certain way . . . For many years, the primary relationship I had with my body was with the mirror.

When I was first introduced to hatha yoga, I began the path or intention of not comparing myself to others. I began to close my eyes and see my true greatness. I began to have a relationship with my body instead of a battle between my head and what I saw in the mirror . . . I could close my eyes to see and not depend upon a mirror to actually affirm or deny whatever my feelings about myself were.

My body just felt so good doing yoga. I was coming into my body and it was an experience I hadn't really felt so far . . . And now I feel more like I love myself and I am so beautiful, and it's not about what I really look like but more about what feels good, and seeing that as real beauty. It makes sense. I think I say that from a place of feeling. I just feel more centered, more connected —like my insides and my external worlds are more meshed than they ever have been. I am more rooted in something that isn't materialistic or part of the game of looking good and winning.

Now I not only know where my shin is but I know how to move it. And this is my thigh and I have known my thighs for a while, but now I know how to move them to create more room in my hips to get to this place where my heart is just singing. It is an ecstatic feeling of joy.

the Divine through the deep acceptance of the way things are. Basic practices such as self-observation and using the body as a vehicle for spiritual transformation sounded exactly like what I had been learning in my hatha yoga studies. At some point I discovered that I was learning tantric philosophy, and how to approach my life from a *genuine* tantric perspective. Unlike the "tantra" of glitz and glitter with sensual oils, dimmed lights and prescribed sexual exercises, tantra as Lee explained it was the non-rejection of all aspects of reality. Tantra "literally means expansion. . . and views all facets of life as natural, but to be transformed and subsumed through spiritual practice."[1] Tantra is a call to embrace all aspects of life as fuel for *sadhana,* or spiritual practice, and as potentially useful to the Divine. Embracing all aspects of life must include all aspects of one's self as well.

When I was eighteen and in treatment for bulimia, my trusted counselor told me that these body image issues would probably follow me around for most of my life. At the time, I was certain that he was wrong about this assessment. I believed that I could do some therapy, get over my issues and put the past behind me. I was so ashamed of my pain and my behavior that I wanted to hide my eating disorder from everyone, including myself. For many years, "looking" recovered from bulimia was actually more important to me that "being" recovered. Because of my refusal to fully accept my issues, my recovery process was compromised. Metaphorically the disease of bulimia was able to dress up in slightly different clothes and continue to live on inside of me, hidden from view.

Many years later, as a counselor at an addiction treatment center, one of my bulimic clients shared that she thought God often gave us the very things from which to recover that we would be the most horrified to have. For example, she was also a hard-core heroin addict, but her first substance addiction was food. In her therapy she often admitted feeling more shame about her bulimia than about anything she had done throughout the time of her heroin use. She didn't

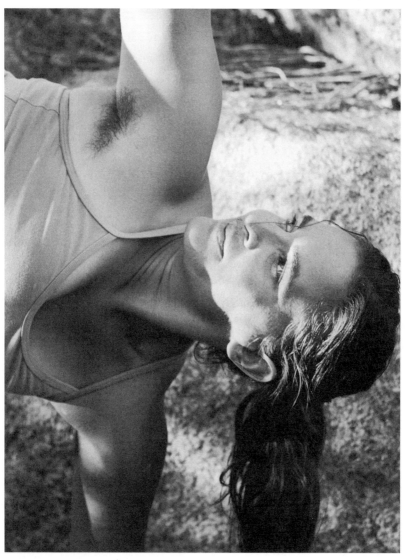

*Ardha chandrasana.* Half moon pose.

want to acknowledge her bulimia—yet accepting her eating disorder was absolutely necessary for her to recover. I could relate to her dilemma.

I have so often hated that I have bulimia. Even the word brought feelings of disgust and shame. In one way, a book about body image and self-esteem that exposes my history of woundedness and self-hatred and focuses on my struggles with bulimia is really the last thing I would ever think was a great idea. I have spent my life cultivating a façade of perfection and of having these issues "all worked out."

To end the war I need to expose the ways that I don't have it all worked out and risk appearing less than perfect. After spending sixteen years battling and/or avoiding these issues, it is an exciting process to begin to make peace with myself, owning the truth of my story in the context of tantric spirituality. Perhaps the things about myself that I have hated the most could actually be useful to other people in terms of service and compassion.

# CHAPTER TWO

# Awakening from the Dream of the Sleeping World

*Unless people learn to differentiate between the essentials*
*and non-essentials, peace will always elude them.*
　　　　　　　　　　　　　　　　　　—B.K.S. Iyengar

Being on a spiritual path, or living according to one's faith, means that a person aligns his/her self to a set of principles and values different than the everyday waking consciousness of our modern culture. I assert that all the variations of consumerism, violence, environmental degradation, human exploitation, broken relationships, psychological dysfunction, betrayal and corruption we witness as commonplace today are all manifestations of a fundamental belief that we are separate from God and therefore separate from each other. Yoga philosophy tells us the truth that we are not separate—that we are part of the One, that our essential nature is divine, pristine and immortal. Yoga philosophy asserts that we are also unaware of that essential truth, dreaming instead a self-centered fantasy that we think is real. Although we walk around and animate a life that seems real, in which we look and act awake, in terms of consciousness potential we are asleep and dreaming. We inhabit the Sleeping World.

The Sleeping World functions according to laws of separation, competition, judgment, domination, submission and division. In terms of body image and self-esteem, the Sleeping

World holds us hostage to ideals for the human body that are unrealistic, often unhealthy, and founded on a lack of respect for our essential worthiness or goodness. The diet industry, the fitness industry, the fashion industry, the cosmetic industry, the entertainment industry, and even the yoga industry, bombard us with images that narrowly define beauty, while setting an unrealistic value on its attainment. An inordinate amount of our time, money, and mental, emotional and spiritual energy are spent in the pursuit of an essentially empty ideal. The Sleeping World is like a big machine that functions to reinforce the myth of separateness, fear, and unworthiness, while convincing us that those meaningless pursuits will relieve our existential suffering. The machine tells us that the suffering we feel is due to conditions such as our looks, our financial status and our psychology.

The Sleeping World hides from us the root cause of our suffering—our mistaken belief that we are separate from God. With the true cause of our suffering hidden and our attention directed toward promised "cures" that actually only perpetuate our suffering, we stay forever trapped in a cycle of illusion and searching. For instance, I believed I wanted to lose weight to be more attractive. The pursuit of weight loss to increase my attractiveness was really motivated by insecurity, and kept me constantly at war with my body. My attention was occupied so I didn't have to question why I felt I needed to be more attractive in the first place. I was thus sheltered from any potential spiritual inquiry—deeper questioning into the nature of reality or even my own psychology.

A sense of pain and longing for union are inherent in the sleeping state itself. The longing is often so subtle and so dampened by the deafening roar of the Sleeping World's clamoring, that we no longer know that there is the greater possibility of conscious life awaiting us. In the spiritual community in which I participate, we often speak of sadhana as a "work on self," or simply, "the Work," a term used by G.I. Gurdjieff, the Russian adept, mystic and teacher who created the "Fourth Way" system of spiritual life.‡ Gurdjieff often used the term, "the Work" when referring to the process by which we evolve consciously in resonance with God or the Absolute.[1] Entering the Work is about exposing the myths of the Sleeping World and learning to listen to the whispers of longing for the real. The Work involves enlarging our focus beyond our ego's limited viewpoint into the larger context of spiritual life. Tantric work is actually about engaging aspects of the dream consciously, with proper guidance, in order to be awakened from the stupor of sleep. Many traditions speak to this when they advise us to "be in the world but not of the world." Lee Lozowick instructs us "to view the world from the perspective of the Work, not to view the Work from the perspective of the world."

Obviously, this instruction is no small task, as we are conditioned to function mechanically—like small machines that are part of a bigger machine. Awakening from the Sleeping World's dream involves having our mechanicality exposed to the light of awareness so that we can begin to chose a new way of relating to the world, to each other and to ourselves. This exposure can be quite shocking and humbling. It can

---

‡Fourth Way: Also known as "the way of the sly man." The methodology of G.I. Gurdjieff, which is said to combine and transcend the three previous ways of spiritual attainment, i.e., the way of the yogi (control of the mind), the way of the fakir (control of the body), and the way of the monk (control of the emotions).

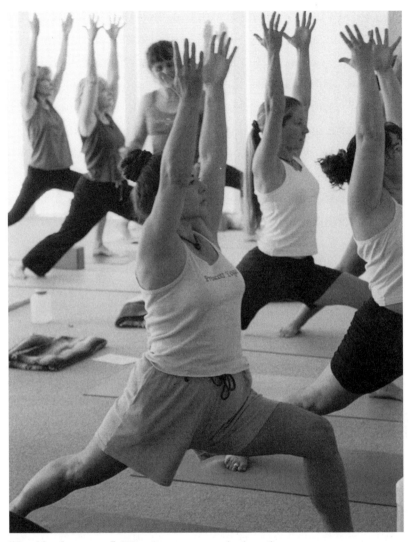

*Virabhadrasana I.* Warrior pose variation 1.

be devastating to realize that even in a culture with its emphasis on individual, independent thought and values, we are still at the mercy of outside forces. A large body of evidence exists that suggests that our beliefs, attitudes and even our preferences are determined predominately by our conditioning—by the Sleeping World.

Most of us are young enough to have been manufactured by advertisers. Our whole value systems are not essential value systems. We have not been allowed to grow up and develop our own ways of relating to the world. Man is a mechanical being anyway— but the quality of the machine has been designed. *Designed!* We are products of a corrupt culture—a culture that is absolutely bereft of any kind of real spirituality. Even among people who have come from the old country the vestiges of traditional life are dying out. There is no real spiritual culture in this country.[2]   —*Lee Lozowick*

The "corrupt culture," the lack of spiritual life and the marketing agencies—all aspects of the Sleeping World—have created a war with the body and the self. The war has many of us playing a game that is unnatural and impossible to win, while calling it "health," "fitness" and "beauty."

Our preferences have slowly been shaped to the point that other people are determining what we see as a desirable and beautiful form for the human body. Marilyn Monroe—one of America's first sex symbols—would probably be considered fat by today's standards or at least very different than the average Hollywood movie star currently in the spotlight. Her dress size, was 12 or 14, which was closer to the average woman's body size than the size 2 or 4 of today's sex symbols. Presently, "the average fashion model weighs 25 percent less than the average woman."[3] One researcher gives this example: "The average American woman is 5'4" tall and weighs 140 pounds. The average fashion model is 5'8" and weighs 117 pounds. Most fashion models are thinner than 98% of American women."[4]

The situation is not improving. In fact, "models get skinnier and skinnier—the average model in 1985 was a size 8, while today the average model is a size 0 or 2."[5]

A research group at Emory University offers the following information:

> The term "body image" has been coined to describe a person's inner sense of satisfaction or dissatisfaction with the physical appearance of his/her body. For most of us, our body image reflects reality: whether we gain or lose a few pounds, achieve muscular definition through exercise or develop "love handles" we generally know it. Our body image is a relatively accurate reflection of our morphology.
>
> But some have body images that are totally out of whack, with perceptions of form and appearance that are extraordinarily distorted. These people are usually women; and although we tend to associate such misperception of one's appearance with anorexia (self-starvation) or bulimia (repeated binging and purging) research now shows that "normal" women suffer from these same body image problems. *In other words, women who have no clinical eating disorder—who appear objectively fine—look in the mirror and see ugliness and fat.*[6] [Italics mine.]

## Diet and Weight: A Family Affair

The general climate of body obsession in the Sleeping World is devastating and the consequences of our national obsession are worsening. Plastic surgery is on the rise, the weight loss industry is booming, and 25 percent of American men

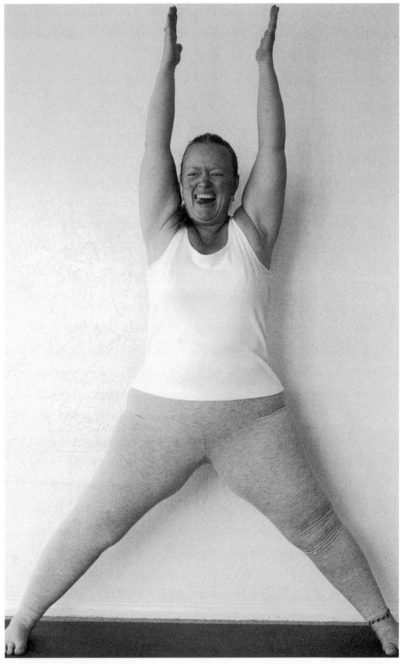

*Urdhva hastasana in prasarita padottanasana.* Arms overhead in wide legged stance.

and 45 percent of American women are on a diet on any given day. Americans spend over $50 billion on dieting and diet-related products each year.[7] The fascination with diet, the addiction to weight loss and the pursuit of the body ideal, has even taken hold of our country's children. A recent survey noted that 42 percent of girls in grades one through three want to be thinner and 81 percent of ten-year-olds are afraid of being fat.[8] In another study, over 75 percent of fourth-grade girls reported that they are "on a diet."[9] A third study concluded that 46 percent of nine-to-eleven-year-olds are "sometimes" or "very often" on diets, and 51 percent of nine-year-old and ten-year-old girls *feel better about themselves* [italics mine] if they are on a diet.[10]

It is no wonder our children are learning these values and behaviors, since 82 percent of the families of these dieting children are "sometimes" or "very often" on diets themselves. Ninety-one percent of women recently surveyed on a college campus had attempted to control their weight through dieting, with 22 percent of those women dieting "often" or "always."[11] Furthermore, more men are suffering from body-image issues and eating disorders than ever before, as are African-American women, who for many years remained free of such symptoms. Some estimates suggest that up to 85 percent of the population suffer from body dissatisfaction.[12] Obviously, the images of the Sleeping World and its standards for the body are pervasive and relentless in their ability to brainwash us into believing their validity.

Much of modern psychological theory focuses on the role the family plays in shaping the personality. In my own work, I have definitely seen the correlation between my upbringing, my bulimia and the way I have treated my body over the years. I think this type of psychological work is important and can be a necessary part of the process of unraveling our conditioning and understanding our behavior. Excellent books have been written on the subject of weight, family dynamics and recovery from eating disorders and various other addictive processes. Few, if any, set "family of origin" dynamics within the context of the Sleeping World's influence. Our parents' thinking and behavior were products of their parents' thinking and behavior. Each generation lives within its own cultural conditioning, and every culture rests firmly in the perception of separation from God. The storylines may change slightly over time to reflect different cultural biases, but the root cause of our suffering is larger than culture and family, although obviously they each play a part in the war with the body.

## Ending the War

The first step of ending the war with the body is to examine the ways that we are attached to the rules of the "body-image game" as defined by the Sleeping World. We can look at why we want to lose those extra five to fifteen pounds or why we think our thighs are too big or too small. We can ask ourselves honestly if twenty pounds, or our cellulite, or the size of our breasts, or the shape of our nose, interferes with our health and our ability to be of service to others. We can examine whether or not the desire to look differently than we do is actually about vanity and seeking approval from the Sleeping World. We can look at the ways our psychological programming has set us up to feel so unlovable that we use our appearance to validate us for the love we feel we are missing. We can explore our existential fear and the ways such fear drives us to control our appearance rather than accept the impermanent, uncertain nature of our very existence. We can begin to honestly face ourselves and the many ways we participate in a war with the body as a way to bolster our self-image and to distract us from what is real.

Obviously obesity can interfere with health in a myriad of ways and I am certainly in favor of people maintaining a weight that feels healthy and functional to them. But, an obsession with perfection based on an unrealistic ideal for the human body and the self-abuse and self-perpetuated violence that we enact on our bodies, minds and spirits as the result of our drive to attain such an ideal is neither healthy nor functional. I suggest that we at least call our own motives into question and begin to align with an ideal that is "real."

As I began my approach to Lee as my teacher, I had a profound confrontation with my own vanity and attachment to the Sleeping World's ideal for my body. One of the rumors I had heard about Lee over the years was that he thought that many women were too thin and would suggest to them that they gain weight. I also noticed as I approached the community of students that many of the women were heavier and rounder than what I thought was acceptable. For almost a year, the fear that Lee would ask me to gain weight was one of the main reasons I did not move closer to him as a teacher. The juxtaposition of my ideals was obvious to me. I saw the essential emptiness of a life spent in the pursuit of the perfect body—the time, the energy, the obsession, and the degree to which the entire game was motivated by vanity had been exposed. Yet, my attachment to the attention and compliments I received for looking thin and "fit" was still quite strong. But there was also my spiritual longing, the guru, and the spiritual community saying that women should be softer, fuller, more essentially feminine and nurturing in order to be more useful and pleasing to the Divine.

These many contradictions were clear and yet terrifying to me, given my history. I had spent over half my life trying to be thin at any cost to conform to the Sleeping World's standard of beauty and to prove to myself and others that I was lovable. However, as the longing in my heart grew for Lee and for what he was offering, as he showed me a love that went beyond my body's appearance, my conditioning and my self-perception, the consideration of weight gain began to diminish in importance. I was able to see and to feel more clearly what was truly real for me, which had nothing to do with the size and shape of my body.

Obviously, my teacher doesn't advocate poor health, obesity, or compulsive overeating either. Nor does he criticize women who are naturally lean and lanky. On the contrary, he is suggesting a natural relationship to the body and to food—a relationship in resonance with the Divine. In such a natural mood the addictions and tensions around food and body image can begin to relax. Ideal weight is simply a function of health. When someone is underweight or overweight the body's energy is spent on adapting to the extreme situation. When the ego is grasping onto a certain image for the body—be it a soft, round image or a lean, muscular image—energy is also wasted on the pursuit of an ideal. Such wasted energy tends to weaken the whole body-mind structure and may encourage various activities ranging from obsessive thinking, self-criticism, and endless comparisons to binging, purging, restricting calories, overeating and over-exercising. Each person must, through a rigorous process of self-observation,

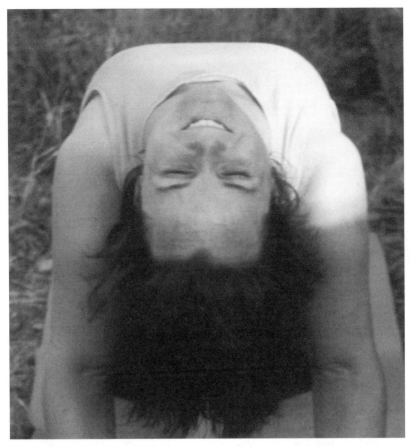

*Ustrasana.* Camel pose.

come to his or her own determination of motives, intention and behavior in regard to these dynamics.

If we are in enough pain about what the war with the body and the self have cost us, then we will be willing to move toward another way of being. We will challenge our belief structures to the degree that we are honest about our pain and exhausted by the struggle. Pain is a great motivator. It gets our attention and tells us that what we are doing may no longer be working. When something hurts badly enough, we are often more willing to make changes.

# Jeannine's Story

*Jeannine, one my African-American students, told me that race adds another dimension to the challenges she faces in her relationship with her body. Originally Jeannine came to yoga to "open spiritual channels" but as she continued her practice, she began to notice her spiritual life merging with her physical form.*

I have definitely had a rocky path with my body. Like most women (I assume) I have struggled to accept and like my body. When I was young, I loved my body and felt comfortable with it. Then as I got older, I started to hate it. There are a lot of factors involved. The first has to do with race. As a child, I lived in many all-white communities, and through prejudice I began to see my-self as less pretty than white girls. I definitely did not hear "Black is Beautiful" from people outside my family. Some of the sadness I experienced from feeling alienated, coupled with family dynam-ics, caused me to not honor my body and to become heavier around puberty. During this time, I developed faster than other

In talking with people for this project, I saw that the more honest someone was about the challenges she faced, the more willing she was to confront the conditioning that shaped her perception. My friend and student Deborah shared with me "that you have to go to hell to heal yourself." And in many ways my research reflected that sentiment. In 12-Step Recovery language, this translates to "hitting bottom." Hitting bottom is what makes us willing to do something different, to try something new. Hitting bottom makes us willing to ask for help. Having exhausted all known avenues, we surrender and open ourselves to the unknown, to the breath of life that only the Divine can bring. For many people, dieting, plastic surgery, over-exercising and self-criti-

girls, having large breasts in my teenage years. From puberty, I always struggled with my weight and with the acceptance of my body. I went into a period where I was bulimic for years.

It's sad but I think that dealing with comparison is the hardest. I know I will never look like a Barbie doll and I don't want to. But that image is everywhere. Our whole society tells us that although you can be uniquely beautiful, the most beautiful women are Barbie dolls. Yoga helps, because the practitioners all have different body types and are all amazing. I love this aspect. At the same time the message of the "perfect type" still comes up. The women with the perfect type always seem to look best in the poses. I know this is not really true, but that's the comparison that always pops up.

The philosophy of yoga (and my spiritual practice) teaches me to let go of my attachment to the way my body looks. What I celebrate most about my body is that it is a temple for my soul. It is this beautiful house that I tend to, but try not to possess or be too attached to. I love that it stores and releases the most amazing currents of energy. I like how joyous it becomes.

cism will actually help to create a feeling of invulnerability to pain. The invulnerability will hold throughout their life and will always be able to distract them from what is real. These people will live forever in the Sleeping World, caught in the mesmerizing web of vanity and the endless pursuit of the unattainable. But for the lucky ones, within the despair of hitting bottom an invitation for a relationship with the Divine will be discovered. When the Sleeping World's message is exposed as a lie, the only option left for some is spiritual life.

My teacher, Lee, frequently speaks about not indulging vanity in the typical ways of the Sleeping World. For what is vanity but the attempt to steel ourselves against our feelings of unworthiness by focusing our attention and aspirations

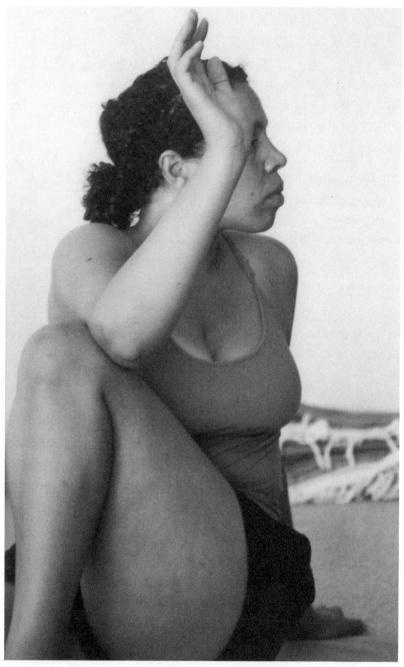

*Ardha matsyendrasana.* Matsyendra's pose. Matsyendra was a sage.

on how we look, what we have and on the endless variations of materialistic, superficial "fixes"? Vanity attaches itself to our feelings of separateness and brokenness—"feelings" that, in truth, are purely phantoms. Since vanity gets its fuel from a myth, why not use our valuable life energy for spiritual work and service rather than for manicuring ourselves or for "looking good." Think about it—if we really knew that the Divine unconditionally loved us, would the concept of a "bad hair day" even make sense? Would we really care so deeply about designer clothes, our complexion, breast size, cellulite, or the number of fat grams we consumed in a day?

I practice keeping myself open to the influence of the grace of God in regard to my body, knowing that with a moderate diet, hatha yoga and an intention to make peace with my body, over time I will settle into my natural weight. I am allowing my longing for God to be bigger and stronger than my longing for a lower weight or a smaller dress size. Lee has suggested to me that the entire notion of "body image" has to go. Simply exchanging a positive body image for a negative body image is not the end of the war, spiritually speaking. Tantric practice demands that we be in relationship with reality, not an image of reality. The imaging itself is part of the problem, as it keeps us tied to the Sleeping World's standards and expectations, focused on the outside appearance of things, rather than the essential nature of reality and the will of the Divine. To surrender one's attachment to an image in our yoga practice, be it positive or negative, creates a practice that moves from the inside out, a practice of peace.

Making peace with the body, practicing yoga from the inside out, is about holding an intention that the very issue of war with the body can be transformed—annihilated through the grace of God in our lives. The yoga scriptures and yoga masters tell us such miracles can happen: "Through the practice of yoga, the impurities of the body and mind are destroyed and the light of knowledge and wisdom dawns."[13] Once we have established an intention, we use our practices to help us endure or celebrate whatever situation we find ourselves in moment to moment. Constant practice, with devotion, over a long period of time helps us to bridge the often-painful gap between our high intentions and our human shortcomings. While we may "know better" we may still constantly find ourselves at the mercy of vanity's tenacious grip, both in our thoughts and in our behavior.

Making peace with the body is a process. Practicing yoga from the inside out happens through disciplined effort over time. Gradually we gain clarity and freedom about what truly motivates us and what is truly most important. This process involves freeing our attention from the war entirely, so that we are able to see, as Werner Erhard puts it, "what is wanted and needed" in every situation. With this insight we are able to serve the people in our lives effectively and to deepen our connection with the Divine. Such service can never be offered when we are consumed with a war on the body. Offering ourselves to this type of selfless service, we often find that the war on the body has realized a cease-fire.

My student, Minnie echoes this sentiment in her own words:

The whole issue or context of body image is a function of our society and the programming and conditioning we've been exposed to, not to mention the unconscious lineage we've adopted from our blood families. It takes a kind of heroic effort to be consciously aware of these subliminal messages and not take them seriously when they arise in our consciousness as "facts."

For example, when a woman "feels" beautiful, she looks beautiful. It may take an unconventional and discriminating eye to notice it. However, when a woman is by nature attractive, yet insecure and neurotic, no amount of acknowledgment from outside will ever convince her of it. Beauty is a function of psychological health, dignity and nobility. When a person knows fundamentally who they are, that is extremely attractive. There is also a personal power and being-presence that radiates outwards usually in the form of generosity of spirit. Happiness sings through the cells of the body and the communication is undeniable.

When I am happy and content, and when I discipline the mind, then "body image" is a ridiculous notion and a waste of my time. The point is to drop the fixation with body image altogether and make other things more important. I believe the fixation and obsession with body image to be a Western affectation that falls naturally by the wayside when there is real suffering that needs our attention.

I am watching a friend die of cancer and that is really helping me to put things into perspective. It is helping me to prioritize the important things in life like service and putting others first. In the face of "real" suffering we can see how silly these preoccupations with the body really are. When a child is really hurting, does it really matter what the shape of our ass is like?[14]

Our bodies and our relationship with our bodies can serve either the machine of the Sleeping World or the Divine. Indulging in behavior that perpetuates the war against the body strengthens the illusion of the Sleeping World, further anchoring its hold on both personal and collective suffering. When hatha yoga is part of our practice of peace, our yoga mats become sacred space. Our time practicing the asanas takes on a deeper meaning and a larger context than the industry of yoga or the machine of Madison Avenue will ever provide. In allowing peace to prevail in our relationship with the body, in learning to live from the inside out, we offer ourselves to the Divine to be used for service. Through our willingness to serve, we create fertile ground in which the seeds of the Divine can grow and bloom into the fruit of true spiritual life and true spiritual culture.

# Kaya Sadhana

*Time was when I despised the body;*
*But then I saw the God within.*
*The body, I realized, is the Lord's temple;*
*And so I began preserving it with care Infinite.*
                    —Bhogar (circa 1600)

*The body is my temple; the asanas are my prayers.*
                    —B.K.S. Iyengar

In tantric work and/or through the practice of hatha yoga, we are involved in *kaya sadhana,* the cultivation of the body as a means for transformation. Lee Lozowick describes the essence of kaya sadhana:

> The mystical, the truly miraculous, is here, and absolutely nowhere else. The doorway is now, not when the presumed obstacle of the body is out of the way. In fact, most people have no idea how literal that description is. We have this illusion that we need to get the body "out of the way" so we can do "real work" or so we can be undisturbed and unhindered by the confusion of emotions and organic urges and desires. But such a circumstance is literally "out of the Way." The Way, that is the spiritual path, the practice of sadhana or of awakening, the Work, is about using what the body makes accessible and possible in all its radiant

glory, in all its profuse confusion, with all its three-centered mess, as the gift of God, as the very—in fact the only—opportunity to advance along the Great Process of Divine Evolution. The body as it is, inclusive of all its elements, levels, gross and subtle, chemical, energetic and "spiritual," is entirely who we are. The body is the body of Work, the body of practice. The body is the Way, and not the "way out" but the Way directly to the heart and soul of God.[1]

Kaya sadhana asserts that we have been given bodies and therefore we can use them for our spiritual growth. Many spiritual teachers over the ages have reminded us that, "We are

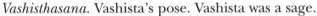

*Vashisthasana.* Vashista's pose. Vashista was a sage.

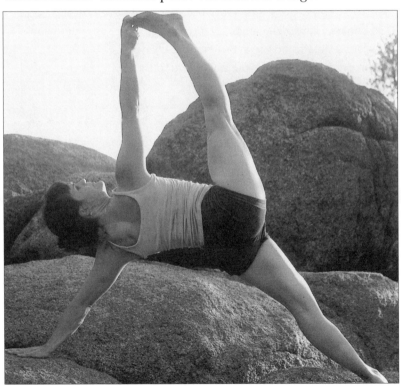

# Cheryl's Story

No matter what size I was, I always felt fat. I was always unhappy. When I would connect with my body, it was never good enough. It seems I have always hated my body.

Even now I still don't look in the mirror at the yoga studio. It is still really hard for me. I keep myself far away and I am grateful when people line up in front of me so I can't see and I don't have to look. So that is the next step for me. But I have come a long way for me—to just show up . . . and to wear spandex and wear smaller shirts that show a little more of my flesh and my body. Those are steps forward for me and I know the mirror will come, but it is definitely intimidating.

I am getting closer and closer to the self-acceptance and the gratitude. Even though I have a fuller body, I am able to do headstands, and handstands and backbends—things that I never perceived I could do! When I looked at yoga magazines and yoga calendars, I didn't see anybody my size. So I just assumed I would never be able to do yoga. But that has changed.

In order to do yoga you really have to be in your body. I could go for a run and be completely out of my body and zoned out. The same thing could happen at the gym. But with yoga it is different. I am sure people can find ways to not be "in the body," but ultimately, if you stay with it, you have got to go within because it is a spiritual practice. If you are opening your body enough then your heart is pounding more and your spirit is becoming more alive. You cannot deny that after a while.

Yoga deepens the relationship with the body. But it goes even deeper than that—I think for me what went deeper was seeing that "I am not my body," and that this practice is a spiritual art. I began to see my body as more of an art form as opposed to just this shell. Once that concept moved through me, I got this feeling , like, "This is my vessel—and there is so much more to me than I knew before. In fact, I'm not even my vessel anymore." Once that relief happened, once that concept moved through, it didn't matter the way I looked.

not human beings having a spiritual experience. We are spiritual beings having a human experience." Many classic yoga scriptures often refer to the body as something we need to transcend, overcome or move beyond. Tantric yoga teaches us to use the body in and for the process of transformation. The body itself is our vehicle. Anusara Yoga teacher Doug Keller explains that "the teaching at stake is that the physical is the portal to the spiritual. Our lesson in this life is to connect with God, the Creator, through His creation; and the only way to experience His creation is in and through the body."[2]

I asked John Friend how hatha yoga, as kaya sadhana, helps us to deepen the relationship with the Self through the body. He replied:

The Self, being the Universal Spirit, is a singular presence. And the body is such a diverse form of that. Through the body we are connecting and seeing that the Universal can be in this little individual package. And then when we move in the body, when we are doing a pose, breathing, and throughout whatever we are doing in the hatha yoga, we can start to find that even as the forms change there is still this singular presence. Even as the body breaks down, even as it ages we can look back and see that we are still that same Self.

I think it happens largely by contrasting. We feel limited in the body and then we start to sense that there is something different than that limited aspect. And that starts to give us the understanding of the Self. Without the limitation we might not have a good contrast and so the understanding of the Universal might not be as deep. That might even explain why God created

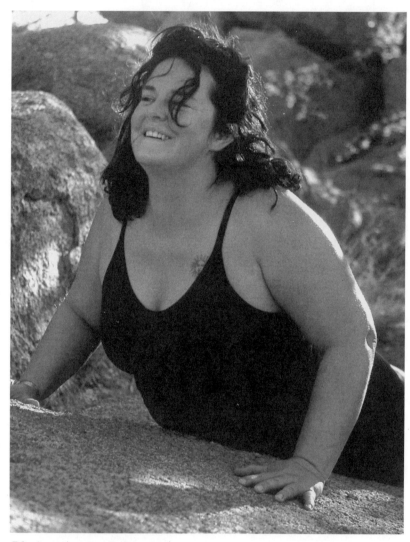

*Bhujangasana.* Cobra pose.

bodies in the first place and why God limits Him- or Herself. Because through that limitation, that contrast, one can really appreciate freedom. And I think that through the body we can gain all the deep insights in the Universe through this little, limited thing that is so corruptible.

As yoga practitioners interested in making peace with the body, we are responsible for practicing in a way that doesn't further corrupt our individual expression of spirit. John continued:

> In doing a certain pose where you might be pushing really hard at a point you are forcing, and you are doing something that is really against the body—so against the body that there is rebellion and injury—it would be like superimposing certain cultural ideals on another nation. And generally war starts out that way—with someone trying to be dominant over someone else. So learning how to back off and learning how different parts of the body are different and different poses are different is important. Also it is important to learn how to work on our bodies to continue to create opening. Not to just say, "Oh my body doesn't like to do that so I am not even going to go there." But to work in a way that you continue to grow. You learn to cultivate contentment and peace with yourself and then in your relationship with others.[3]

If the body is truly the vehicle for God realization, it is logical and necessary that in our practice of kaya sadhana we develop our ability to see the body as holy. But we cannot jump from a war with the body to a perspective that simply claims "the body is our temple." We must begin with the practice of making peace, over time aligning our behavior with our intention to offer peace. Through our various practices we treat the body with the love and respect it deserves as our means for spiritual transformation.

A friend recently shared with me an excerpt from one of her journals, which speaks about her process of making peace with her body within the context of kaya sadhana and life with a spiritual master:

> When I was in junior high and high school, I had a severe case of acne. The pain and torment I went through each time I looked at myself in the mirror was devastating. I spent the first few years with a morning regime that took hours. First I would look at myself with disgust and horror. Most days I would cry. Then I would take my medicated soap out of its box and proceed to scrub. And I mean scrub. I think I used everything short of steel wool on my face desperately trying to erase my ugly condition. Then I would cake on every conceivable brand of cover up available from medications to the greasiest pancake make-up money could buy. Then in high school I began to go to a dermatologist. I will spare the description of the nightmares of that experience. I had not one date all those years. I spent my weekend evenings at home listening to records and watching TV. After all, who would want to go out with a monster?

> For thousands of other women, the same type of obsession and victimization has caused severe sexual frigidity. For others, grotesque sexual promiscuity and prostitution. For some women it has meant years of addictions such as the vicious amphetamine/barbiturate cycle. And for others it has triggered a vast array of eating disorders, the most severe being anorexia and bulimia. There are women who are lit-

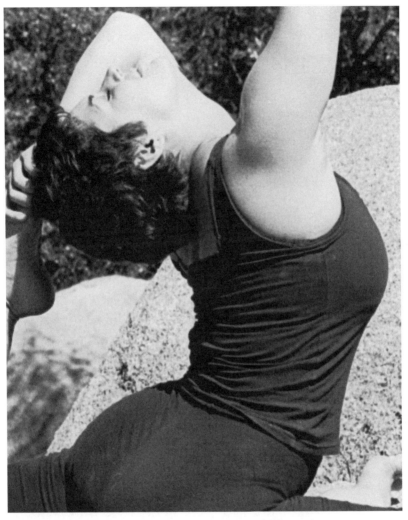

*Eka pada rajakapotasana I.* One leg royal king pigeon pose, variation 1.

erally starving themselves to death due to a psychotic fear of weight gain. Now there are reports of women who are doing the same thing with aerobics, triathlons, and running. The cure rate for anorexia is one of the lowest of all psychosomatic disorders. Self-starvation, slow suicide, failure to thrive; triggered by pressure from society and family to be successful, popular, and THIN. The personal anguish and torture I have gone through and witnessed in close friends is truly heartbreaking.

And what lies at the root of all this? Is our society so decadent, are our ideals so distorted and is the fear of isolation and being unloved so fantastic that women are literally being forced to starve themselves to death rather than face some possible rejection or the fate of being single at 35 or 40? Do some of us truly believe that we are so unworthy of love because we are not perfect cover girls or Playboy bunnies that we would rather throw up every morsel of nourishment we ingest rather than be responsible for that love?

As women in the company of a spiritual master we have been given the opportunity to turn our conditioned, distorted views of our bodies—complete with wrinkles, cellulite, pimples, scars and graying hair—into accepting and loving views of ourselves as potential devotees who can be as vibrant, juicy, voluptuous, fleshy, and radiant as any of Krishna's gopis were.[‡] We have an opportunity for our "neurosis to transcend itself in love."[‡‡] I would say that this is quite an

---

[‡]In Hindu mythology, Krishna had many devotees who were cow-herds, the *gopis* and *gopas*. In one legend he danced with 10,000 gopis on one night; vibrant, beautiful women who sought and experienced ecstatic union with him, their Beloved. The term "gopi" has become synonymous with ecstatic devotee.

[‡‡]Refers to a principle described by Lee Lozowick. To have neurosis transcend itself in love is to have the power of love and the influence of the Divine become bigger than the influence and power of neurotic tendency.

extraordinary consideration. In light of this consideration, it seems it would be worth our while as women in spiritual work to think about this when we look in the mirror rather than whatever it is we have been conditioned to think about that reflection.[4]

For those of us who have been at war with the body, kaya sadhana has to do with encountering our various body-related judgments and neurosis. We must practice embodiment as a part of our path toward enlightenment. To say that the body is a vehicle for transformation, and then not address the body hatred or the violence we enact upon the sacred ground of the body, is certainly a contradiction. We must face ourselves honestly.

More important, however, than identifying the myriad ways that our hatred or our body-oriented neurosis manifests, is the possibility of neurosis being transformed into love. The practice of hatha yoga opens us to such a possibility by helping us to experience love, joy and ecstasy in the body.

In an article entitled "Yoga: A Path of Optimization," yoga teacher Ria Roamno reflects:

> There is a passage in the *I Ching* (the *Book of Changes*, an ancient system of divination) that says, "You cannot fight the devil directly. When you do you tend to become the devil that you are fighting." Instead the Chinese Oracle recommends that you "fight the devil by emphasizing what is good and allowing that to replace the darkness."[5]

Practicing hatha yoga with the intention of making peace isn't a set of rule-based procedures that we employ mechanically in our practices. Practicing yoga from the inside out, as a practice of peace, is a context we hold for ourselves in which we allow ourselves to open to what is greater than our darkness. Hatha yoga can give us the opportunity to build on what is good and whole within ourselves, rather than focusing our attention solely on our darkness and neurosis.

One of the great gifts of hatha yoga is that it focuses our attention internally, on the sensations of the body rather than on its appearance. By changing where we focus our attention, hatha yoga helps to shift our context for how we experience the body, and in many cases how we experience the world around us. Instead of a battlefield, the body becomes a vehicle for greater awareness, for spiritual practice, self-expression and celebration. The body actually becomes our salvation, our means of true authenticity and spiritual transformation.

# CHAPTER FOUR

# *Paying Attention*

Imagine this scenario: You are tired and stressed out after work. You are racing down the highway to get to your yoga class, driving twenty-five mph over the speed limit. You honk at drivers in your way and then tailgate someone for the last mile of the drive, silently urging them to get on with it. Once there, you race up the stairs to your class and rush into the room, oblivious to the fact that class has started, and throw down your yoga mat. In a huff, you sit down and attempt to join in. The class has been warming up for several minutes but you skip that part, considering it unnecessary. Instead, you proceed to stretch to your maximum, thinking that "more is better," meanwhile forgetting about your hip that tends to go out of joint, the wrist pain you have been having and the fact that you aren't supposed to practice inverted postures because you have your period. When the instructor says to use the mirror to assess your alignment, you notice the cellulite on your thighs and decide to skip dinner. When the instructor directs you to look at your feet, you look at your worn out pedicure and think how horrible your feet look, mentally reviewing your schedule for when you could get to the salon. Since you are so busy, you decide to skip the final relaxation pose, *sivasana,* and leave early. You think to yourself, "What is so important about just lying there anyway?"

While the example above is extreme, the point is that one can certainly practice yoga in a way that is inattentive, and this lack of attention can be neglectful or even violent. To practice with intention would yield quite a different scenario: You carefully roll out your mat acknowledging that this is a time of spiritual practice—a time for honoring your body and your self. You report your injuries and limitations to your teacher and work carefully throughout the practice. When asked to use the mirror to assess your form, you look objectively at the alignment of your structure and look with kindness on your body, reminding yourself that you are fine exactly as you are. Looking at your feet you clearly observe their placement and the action of the arches. When you feel pain, you look into it. You ask yourself if it is joint pain, muscular teaching or just intense sensation? Can you still breathe fully even in the intensity? If not, you look for a new alignment or modification. If you can still breathe, you assess your psychological state, asking yourself if it would be okay to stay in the intensity or be better in that moment to release the pose? With each inhalation you practice expanding the heart and with each exhalation you offer out your prayers and gifts. You allow the poses to shine with heartfelt qualities of the spirit, and you remind yourself that you are doing great!

To create peace we must see the war we wage with stark clarity and objectivity. We must learn the intricacies of the ways we sabotage our own efforts. Setting the intention for hatha yoga to be a practice of peace means making an ongoing commitment to such self-observation. "Self-observation is about bringing an honesty and depth of clarity to manifestations, motivations and behaviors. It means to see objectively from an observer's point of view without justifying, rationalizing, projecting, implying or excusing anything, and obviously without any feelings of pride, vanity, guilt or shame as a result of what we observe in ourselves."[1]

The hatha yoga practitioner uses the body as the vehicle of consciousness, as the terrain for practice, exploration and observation. To practice self-observation in hatha yoga we use the asanas to witness the sensations of the body, the thoughts of the mind, the feelings of the heart, and the majestic simplicity of the spirit. Over time, a deeper relationship with the body and the self emerges because of the attention that has been paid to the integration of the body, mind and spirit. Paying attention to people is one of the best ways to show them that we love and care for them. In the practice of hatha yoga we can hone our ability to pay attention to the physical alignment of the body in space, our attitudinal alignment with our heart's desire and the spiritual alignment we have with the Divine. By paying attention to ourselves through self-observation in our yoga practice we show ourselves that we are worthy of our own attention, making our practice into an act of love. In this spirit of love, yoga can become an offering of peace.

When we begin to pay attention we may be shocked by the steady barrage of criticism and judgment we have about our body—it is too big, too small, too wrinkled, too pale, too short, too tall, too stiff. We may observe that we constantly compare ourselves to others—they know more, can do more, look better, get more attention, are prettier, taller, smaller, thinner, stronger and more flexible. The practice of self-observation asks us to observe ourselves *without judgment,* and so we notice when we are judging ourselves but we do not indulge in judging ourselves about our judgments. Instead we

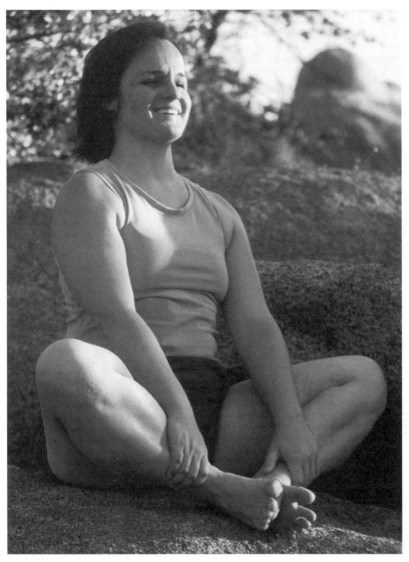

*Badha konasana.* Bound angle pose.

just notice that judgment is arising. We simply observe what is happening in the moment.

It is important to remember that in the process of self-observation we do not give equal weight to all that surfaces from within. While tantric philosophy suggests that all aspects of life are Divine, it does not suggest that all aspects are equal. Tantric practice asks us to make choices, to make meaningful distinctions between external and internal manifestations, based on the spiritual values and principles with which we are aligned. Although we notice everything that arises with objectivity and without judgment, we also practice discernment in order to assess which of our internal mechanisms serve our work and which of these patterns hinder our growth and development. This discernment function is a natural result of the practice of paying attention through self-observation and not a muscled effort of forced personal change. An honest self-review will reveal the choices we have to make in what to accentuate in ourselves and what to minimize.

## Paying Attention to the Body

*Do not fight the body . . . do not kill the instinct of the body for the glory of the pose. Do not look at your body like a stranger, but adopt a friendly approach towards it. Watch it, listen to it, observe its needs, its requests, and even have fun. Play with it as children do, sometimes it becomes very alert and swift.*

*To be sensitive is to be alive.*
        —Vanda Scaravelli, *Awakening the Spine*

Often the relationship we have with the body is one of extremes. People commonly ignore the needs of the body, mindlessly dragging themselves through the day, out of touch with their natural rhythms and needs. For example, we eat when we are not hungry or often diet to the point of being hungry all the time. Many of us have no reliable sensor of "full" and often overfeed our bodies beyond what they require to function, which leads to weight gain, physical sluggishness and emotional numbness. When we are tired, we may drink coffee rather than rest. We wear fashionable shoes that distort the feet and create postural difficulties and discomfort throughout the body. In exercise, some of us learn to ignore pain and to push past our natural limits, while others are so afraid of exertion that they never make healthy demands on their bodies and thus fail to thrive.

In the practice of yoga we develop a set of communication skills that deepen our ability to pay attention—to speak, to listen and to respond to the sensations of the body. This practice of communicating with the body begins to fuse the body and the mind, creating union, or "yoga." The practice of aligning the physical body according to biomechanical principles is often simply referred to as "alignment." This practice involves implementing specific instructions about the optimal placement of the body in the different yoga poses so as to increase mobility, decrease the risk of injury and to create poses that have both freedom and stability. The study of alignment in asana and the practice of aligning the physical structure help to strengthen this union, allowing us to practice from the inside out and to confront the stereotypes of the Sleeping World that for so long have determined our body image. Aligning a pose is not only physical—it actually happens "on many different levels, from the gross outer form to the highly refined inner quality."[2]

In the physical domain, the study of alignment focuses our attention on the physical structure in an objective, no-nonsense way. We begin to learn about the body, focusing more on anatomy and physiology than on cosmetics and appearance. We learn the details of optimal alignment and learn how to create greater mobility and ease. We learn about

## Sarah's Story

I don't think that I even had much of an awareness of my body until I was about 15 or 16. If I did it was very external—what I was wearing—clothes, makeup, etc. When I was in high school I definitely had issues that were probably very normal for that age. I was always on some crazy diet like eating only rice cakes and carrot juice. Or I wouldn't eat all day. Thinking of those times now makes my body want to curl up—I would go for months that way.

I get frustrated with my weight and with food, and more recently I have been having symptoms like yeast infections, kidney infections and intestinal problems. These things are always pulling me back to my body and to food. I think, "Why can't I just eat a piece of cake or two on somebody's birthday?"

I wish I could get to a point where my body voice or intelligence was louder than my mind. That is extremely out of balance most of the time. My therapist asks me, "What is out of control in your life and what can you pull back into control in your life instead of focusing on your body?" But that is a hard thing to think about when you are in a cycle of hating your body—it's hard to think about what feels out of control when everything feels simultaneously fine and out of control.

In the ninety minutes of yoga class I have criticizing thoughts about my body, but it seems like I don't have time to focus on them. So in class, they are fleeting—they come and they leave.

muscles and how they act upon our skeleton and we learn to see our body through a lens of discerning objectivity, rather than by subjective, culturally-defined standards of beauty. We begin to place our attention on the body in a way that values strength, flexibility, range of motion, ease of movement and sensitivity. In order to apply principles of proper alignment, we learn a new way to see the body. Then we learn to enter into the body itself with our awareness and intention.

When I am not in yoga, and I am in that process of criticism, I get dragged down into the negativity.

Yoga sometimes seems to amplify my criticizing. Doing a position, I often get frustrated, or look at myself in the mirror and think I look fat. But I think setting my intention at the beginning of yoga and affirming why I am doing it and coming back to that is helpful. I am finding a way to soften a little bit to those voices inside.

I am wearing tight pants and that is a huge risk for me. I will notice bulges and I can think to myself, "I am okay with that." I get frustrated doing hip openings but in my reaffirming that I am here to do yoga, I can just "be with" the frustration.

Yoga for me is about developing a softness towards myself emotionally, because I am harsh. I think it is quieting that part of myself. I can be angry and pissed off and let it go and not feel such an attachment to it. It is okay if I can't get into a certain position today because I can always try tomorrow.

I am addicted to yoga and I don't really know why I don't think about what I am going to do when I get there—I just get there. My practice is just to get to yoga. Yoga is a whole new experience. You just come, and whatever unfolds, unfolds. I am able to cry at different times or to laugh. We end up laughing a lot and that feels really good. And there are times when I come when I am a total grump but I still follow the positions. I love the awareness that comes with yoga.

In the course of studying alignment-oriented methods of hatha yoga we are often asked to assess unknown and even seemingly obscure parts of the body. We are asked to move these parts of the body in ways that are counter to our habitual patterns and require skill. Although we hope to gain control and mastery over these areas and movements, it is the very process of going within, not the perfection of the pose, which paves the way to peace with the body.

Probing these unknown areas and moving in these unfamiliar ways strengthens our relationship with the body and increases our ability to move from the inside out as we practice. For instance, one of the instructions often given in Anusara Yoga classes is to "lift or inflate the kidneys." In other classes, I have even been instructed to "lift the skin above the kidneys up the back and to move the skin below the kidneys down the back." To the average person, such an instruction is not only obscure but also meaningless and impossible to execute. It is not surprising then, that many people don't even attempt to follow such instructions. However, over time we learn that instructions dealing with the area of the kidneys(the middle back) move our awareness more deeply into what is often called "the back body."

The back body is representative of the unconscious; the collective rather than the individual; of the things unseen that "back us up" and provide support for our individual efforts. Additionally, the area of the kidneys creates a bridge between the lower and upper halves of the body and serves to integrate the forces in life that lift us up with those that anchor and ground us to the earth. Suddenly such an instruction as "move more into your kidneys" has a meaning that is deeper than simply lengthening the spine or trying to do the impossible. When we implement the instruction to "move into the back body" we are not only rewarded with a longer spine and stronger experience of our physical strength but we are also more aware of our personal connection with Divine support and the support of the community. We may feel that suddenly we have a "backbone" and that we are surer of ourselves. Because we are trusting in *things unseen* for support, we are training ourselves to be less seduced by the distractions that we do see out in front of us that so often clamor for our attention.

This journey into the "back body" is one more aspect of the process of making peace with the body. When we practice in such a manner, we are literally transforming the asana practice into an offering, into a devotional prayer, where the asanas physicalize our intention, creating a union of mind and body.

## Paying Attention to the Mind

*Spiritual knowledge grows from the unionof the head and the heart.* —B.K.S. Iyengar

In paying attention to the mind we can observe our mental outlook and notice without judgment the tone with which we practice. Through self-observation we become aware of the ways we are at war with the body. As we clearly observe the consequences of such self-inflicted violence and begin to choose peace, we are encouraged to stay mindful and committed to our intention, carefully redirecting our thoughts toward acceptance throughout our practice.

When we practice yoga we actually give the mind something to focus on in the here and now. We discipline the mind to be in the present moment. In this way yoga is a meditation and aligns itself with the first of Patanjali's *Yoga Sutras:* "Now let us come together to practice yoga." *Now* is the time when we practice yoga. We are in the moment as we watch what our breath is doing; we are in the moment as we practice our alignment principles; we are in the moment as we observe our judgments and as we lovingly guide ourselves back to our intention for making peace. Now is what we have.[3]

The importance of being in the moment was reinforced for me when I taught yoga to a friend who has cancer. In

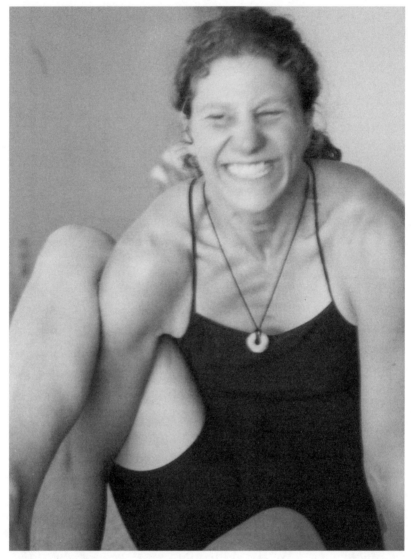

*Eka hasta bhujasana.* One arm squeezing pose.

dealing with her disease over the last several years, she experienced diminished physical strength. She asked me to show her some yoga stretches as her other exercises were proving too strenuous. As we worked to find her limits and to identify poses and modifications that she could do without pain,

I was reminded of some of the most essential aspects of hatha yoga such as going inward and growing more mindful with each breath. Using the asanas we align the mind, the body and the spirit in the present moment, becoming more aware of what we find inside ourselves right now.

This experience with my friend confronted me with the fact that I am often distracted from these fundamental principles of practice by fancy poses, by strong students who are "getting better" at yoga, and by my own drive to achieve more. My friend and I were not working together to find ways for her to "get better" or "to make progress." Chances are she is not going to be able to do difficult poses any time in her future. Instead, we were working together to find some way to bring her into the present moment, to deepen her relationship with her body in a way that was empowering and mindful. In her gentle, modified practice she was coming into her body and listening for what felt beneficial and what felt detrimental. She was aligning with the practice of making peace with the body.

My friend was also able to observe the emotions that surfaced as she practiced her yoga. She noted her feelings of discouragement and loss in the deterioration of her physical body and energy level, not only from her cancer but also from radiation and chemotherapy. Continued yoga practice can offer her an opportunity to see and grieve her losses honestly and to focus on what she *could* do rather than on what she couldn't. As her illness progresses, her yoga practice might simply become watching her breath or observing the pain in her body. It will involve managing her "mind chatter" as her ability to care for herself diminishes and her reliance on her caregivers increases. Her yoga practice of peace will be an attempt to surrender control while maintaining a sense of humor, dignity, self-respect and trust in God. Regardless of the form that her specific practice takes over time, my friend can use the principles of hatha yoga to offer peace to herself and to offer the efforts of her practice to the Divine. I have the opportunity to apply these insights to my own practice of peace as well.

No matter what the state of the physical body, we can each come more fully to the present moment. The perspective of yoga as a pathway "in" can permeate our journey and confront our perfectionist strivings that steer us away from life just as it is. With each breath, with each pose, we can practice the yoga of "be here now." And now. And now. Like pearls strung together to make a beautiful necklace, the moments we stay conscious and present will string together to form our lives and our practices. In the beauty, wonder and simplicity of the moment, there is less room for the endless projections of self-hatred, body-oriented criticism and fear-based judgment.

## Paying Attention to the Emotions

*It is the work of the spiritual student to feel. And it is his work to begin to allow the false masks and suits of armors that surround crystallized ways of behavior and relationship to crumble so that the Divine Influence of his spiritual teacher may resurrect true being and full feeling in the place of emptiness and constricted life.*

—Lee Lozowick

When we approach yoga in a mindful way, we become aware of the emotional processes that take place during the practice. My experience has shown me that hatha yoga is a very emotional practice, often transporting the practitioner to states of revelatory ecstasy as well as into the swamps of human fear, insecurity, anger and loneliness. One moment we are in a yoga pose listening to an instruction, the next moment we are flooded with feelings of shame, guilt or sadness.

Unpleasant emotions often arise that are linked to our body-history. As we assume a posture, perhaps our instructor adjusts us in a way that hurts or speaks to us harshly and we are immediately reminded of past abusers who also spoke to us in harsh tones. Or perhaps the body is simply releasing feelings and stored emotions. For instance, at this stage in my practice when I find myself slightly injured or hurting in a pose, in a way that feels like a strain, my eyes flood with tears. It is as if I am magnetically pulled back to the recognition of how much pain I have endured in my body throughout my life. When these tears arise, I observe them without judgment or criticism. I do my best to honor my process without indulging in any sentiments of victimization or blame. I inquire about whether I need to adjust my position and realign my body more accurately, or if I simply need to allow my emotions to run their own course.

Interestingly, unpleasant emotions rarely surface initially with stark objectivity. Most often they surface attached to our personal storylines or our projections about how we are not good enough, how we are misunderstood, how we are always abused or yelled at or ignored, how teachers are all phonies and cannot be trusted, how we are not thin enough, or how we never get any attention. It is very important to understand that the mind and the emotions are intimately linked, and to distinguish between the raw feeling that is being released from the body and the negative self-talk that creates emotions of unworthiness, victimization, doubt and shame.

Recently I attended a workshop where the instructor used a loud tone of voice as he taught. He commanded me to deepen my pose—one that was painful for me. "More," he boomed several times, to which I replied, "I am trying!" My knee began aching and I noticed my sadness arising. He yelled, "You are not *trying* anything but my patience!" Immediately tears welled up. I felt shame, anger and sadness. And then I thought of my spiritual teacher, Lee. I prayed to be able to see the situation objectively. In the next moment, the instructor came over to me and began working with me to bring my pose into better alignment. I let the tears flow but I also began to feel his compassion that is always present for me even in his gruff manner. I felt his commitment to helping me in that moment and over the last several years, and I saw how his comment that I was trying his patience wasn't personal, even though he said it to me and even though it had hurt my feelings. I understood that the fear I was experiencing was about my body approaching a limit. My shame was about what I was projecting that other people in the room might be thinking about me. My sadness was about the past and my history with my body, not about the way I was practicing in the moment.

My initial response to this instructor's teaching that night was to feel hurt and to become angry. Justified in my anger and feeling resentful, I could have decided to leave the workshop and never study with this teacher again—a pattern that is common for me. It boils down to "checking out," leaving a relationship, and leaving the moment. By practicing self-observation and objectivity rather than indulgence of my feeling state, and by invoking the presence of my teacher, I reached a new level of insight about my practice and about

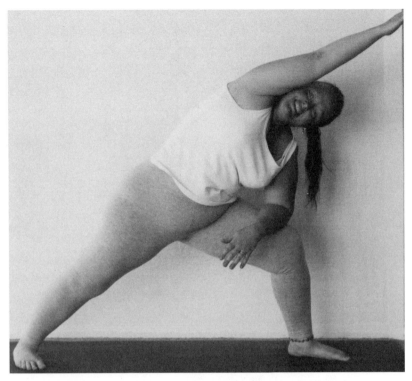

*Parsvakonasana variation.* Side angle pose variation.

how best to continue to work with this yoga instructor. I discovered that I could honor my feelings and my body, and, at the same time, cultivate detachment in regard to a situation that triggers my outdated beliefs. I realized that to continue advancing in my practice I would need to develop a new way of being in my body—a way of being with intense physical sensations that could be separated from my history of abuse and neglect.

Moving into a deeper relationship with my pain requires a more refined dimension of the practice of peace—beyond simply "stopping whenever something hurts" a phrase that describes my initial approach to pain. There is a natural pain that is healthy and associated with opening areas of the body that

## *Minnie's Story*

The history is an unhappy one, yet, I believe, not uncommon. Mood swings and different perceptions of how I have appeared, unfortunately overrode how I *actually* felt in my body. Vanity and obsessive/compulsive behavior with food, drugs and alcohol permeated my teenage years. And always I maintained an attitude that I was ashamed of my physical form.

One of the key benefits that my spiritual teacher had expressed in the practice of daily exercise has to do with the breath. With exercise I usually felt emotionally and mentally cleaned out. I call it a way of "taking out the garbage." However, with the practice of yoga I recognize a more subtle relationship at play.

Besides overcoming the daily resistance I have to actually practicing yoga, I notice that I am forced to feel what is going on for me at deeper levels—linked to the habitual thought patterns that are part of that circuitry. There are parts of my body that have been energetically dormant due to things like poor posture, poor eating habits—dormant in the sense that there have been revealed to me (through yoga practice) many small muscles that I have simply not exercised or used most of my life.

Even though my experimentation with other forms of exercise has always been exhilarating and fulfilling, I have somehow sensed that the work could go more deeply. I had made small inroads but never actually shifted context with these issues and relationship to my body. This is the gift of yoga.

It's not a matter of what others think about how I look. It comes from a less superficial sense of how I feel. When I feel grateful for my life there is radiance that communicates and when that happens I feel really full and juicy and alive.

have been closed for many years. A different quality of pain results from unconsciously forcing the body past its limits. There are also various emotional pains that may surface as we practice. Yoga as a path of peace calls for me to discern among these different types, acknowledging them all, but understanding that different pain may call for different responses.

Yoga is meant to help us fuse the body with the mind, the mind with the soul, and the individual self with the universal self. Each person who practices yoga long enough will come to face themselves emotionally time and again in the pursuit and practice of this union. When feelings and emotions surface in our practice we can allow them to come into the light of our acceptance. We don't always have to stop our practice session, but we can learn to "be *with* our feelings" which is really quite different from "going into our feelings." Being with our feelings involves self-observation and looking upon the experience of the feelings with detached interest and clarity. Going into our feelings would mean losing perspective and allowing the emotional state to take over the process of objective observation. For instance, when sadness shows up, we can allow the tears to follow their natural course while continuing to perform our asanas, paying attention to our breath and to our internal self-talk. If anger surfaces, we allow it into the light of awareness yet take care not to turn the anger against ourselves by hardening in our poses or using it to fuel an over-efforted practice.

Energetically, emotions are quite powerful. Paying attention to our emotions is a dynamic way of honoring ourselves and keeping the treaty of peace with the body. Many of our war-oriented behaviors stem from the attempt to numb ourselves against reality and the pain of suffering—which may be personal or transpersonal. The feelings we attempt not to feel will run the gamut from despair to elation. (My opinion is that joy is one of the most suppressed feelings around.) Regardless of the emotion or its source, practicing yoga from the inside out asks us to stay present to our feelings in an authentic way. Hatha yoga, because it brings us into the body and into the moment and also has the ability to release stored feelings from the body tissue itself, becomes an invaluable tool for not only observing our feelings but for learning a way to express and honor them. By aligning our emotional expression with our practice of hatha yoga as a peace offering, we are extending the practice of peace beyond the body. We thus experience a union, a yoga that reveals to us the true interconnectedness of the body, the mind and the spirit.

## Paying Attention to the Spirit— Aligning the Human

*As we practice we are literally aligning ourselves bodily to the Great Process of Divine Evolution.*

—Lee Lozowick

The art of practicing with alignment is multi-dimensional. Alignment can be philosophical, emotional, physical, and/or intentional. Proper alignment can mean the difference between the breakdown and the breakthrough of the practitioner. When the physical body is aligned correctly, an asana will rehabilitate the body and help it to function more easefully. Proper alignment will heal injuries, open the body in new ways and allow the practitioner to practice more difficult poses with grace and freedom. Breakthrough! When poses are practiced with the body even slightly off of ideal alignment, the body will deteriorate over time. Breakdown.

When the mind is aligned to the present moment during the practice of asana, the mind will clear and experience focused awareness. When the mind is aligned with the practitioner's intention, the mind can help serve a transformational

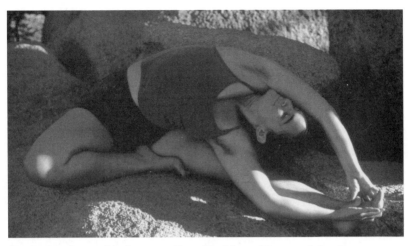

*Parivritta janu shirshasana.* Revolved head beyond the knee pose.

purpose rather than create the havoc of undisciplined thought. Breakthrough! When the mind is aligned with the Sleeping World and its values . . . when the mind is seeing the body through the eyes of the world and not through the eyes of the Work . . . we are at war. Breakdown.

In the spiritual domain, the practice of alignment gives us the opportunity to align ourselves with the Divine, to our spiritual teacher or guru, thereby infusing our practice with the sacred. Such alignment can be called *resonance.* When we practice our yoga in a way that is resonant to the Divine, that honors our sense of the sacred, we are practicing our yoga as an offering of peace. Breakthrough! To disregard the Divine, to practice yoga that is harsh, critical, violent and motivated by vanity, striving and competition, we are out of resonance. We are at war. Breakdown.

For much of my life, exercise was one of my strongest weapons in the war with my body. By over-exercising, refusing to rest appropriately, and obsessing about my shortcomings constantly throughout a workout, I perpetuated the war against my body. To invoke the sacred in an apparently physical regime such as hatha yoga, to invite God into my practice, demands that I practice differently than my history has taught me. If my intention is to offer peace, and my understanding is that yoga can lift some of the veils that block me from experiencing the ever-present reality of grace, then to practice with harsh criticism and violence is truly out of spiritual alignment. To practice yoga with proper spiritual alignment requires me to soften, to relax and to listen to my body with compassion and sensitivity; to practice from the inside out.

When I practice yoga, I consciously invoke the presence of my spiritual master and the lineage in which he teaches to guide me during my practice. I intend that my yoga practice is a time to experience his benediction more fully. I understand that grace is always present, constantly showering upon me, and I use my yoga practice to open myself more fully to the awareness of such blessings. It is the same way in spiritual life: when we are aligned to the teaching, to a teacher and/or to the sangha (practitioners), we find ourselves in a certain flow within a particular current of grace. When we are even slightly out of alignment with our chosen path, there is unnecessary suffering. Just as an asana performed out of alignment will cause pain and a properly aligned asana will heal, a life lived out of spiritual alignment will cause suffering whereas a spiritually-aligned life will lead to freedom and true happiness.

In spiritual life we are asked to align the human with the Divine, to fuse the mundane with the sacred. Through hatha yoga we can align our physical structure with its highest potential, we can align our mental structures with our Divine intentions, and fully awaken to our true nature. We can align with grace.

# Opening the Heart: Uncovering and Expressing Our True Nature

*Softness, vulnerability, spontaneity, kindness, goodness,
compassion, real pride, dignity are inherent in our
natural, primary condition.*

—Lee Lozowick

In the process of making peace with the body, we begin
with the idea that inherent in the ground of our being is a
natural state that, in my tradition, is called "organic innocence." In this state a "natural ecstasy" manifests physically,
mentally, and emotionally. Through our sadhana, we are
aligning ourselves with this natural state of organic innocence, rather than with the Sleeping World's ideals and standards. For human beings to function from organic
innocence is to live from the instinctual knowledge of the
body, because the body is innately wise.[1]

Many different spiritual traditions speak to a similar concept. *Advaita vedanta* master,‡ Arnaud Desjardins, reminds
us in his teacher's words "that every single being has intrinsic
dignity and intrinsic nobility."[2] Chögyam Trungpa Rinpoche,
a master of Tibetan Buddhism, called this same state "basic
goodness," saying:

‡Advaita vedanta: The doctrine of non-dualism, which proposes that the
Absolute Reality and the individual soul are identical in their transcen-
dantal nature.

It's not just an arbitrary idea that the world is good, but it is good because we can experience its goodness. We can experience our world as healthy and straight-forward, direct and real, because our basic nature is to go along with the goodness of the situation. The human potential for intelligence and dignity is at-tuned to experiencing the brilliance of the bright blue sky, the freshness of green fields and the beauty of the trees and mountains. We have an actual con-nection to reality that can wake us up and make us feel basically, fundamentally good.[3]

For many of us who have been brought up believing that we are fundamentally flawed and undeserving of love, it can sound scary to discuss uncovering and expressing our true na-ture. Our families, teachers, and even our religions have told us how unworthy we are. Within Christianity we learn that we are born sinners. We are born with original sin. It is really no surprise that from such a starting point we would enter into a destructive relationship with the body and the self. With the core belief that we are born bad or wrong, it is logical to make choices that would prove such a belief true.

If we remain aligned to our intention to practice hatha yoga from the inside out, as a practice of peace with the body, we will honestly face the many manifestations of our belief in original sin, which is nothing other than our mistaken no-tion that we are separate from God. We will face our negative thoughts about ourselves and about others, our destructive patterns and the many ways we create and perpetuate vio-lence with the self. If we persevere in our intention to make peace, we will also practice focusing on love, rather than on our neurosis. We will begin to uncover the beauty of our open hearts instead of only demons, darkness and pain. We will begin to uncover our basic goodness and to experience ourselves within a context of greatness and grace. We are more than our pain, our suffering and our belief that we are separate from God and from each other.

In making peace with the body, we use the idea of basic goodness to give us courage in facing ourselves. If we understand that basic goodness is our very nature, then when what is arising from within is difficult to accept, we can return to the notions of intrinsic dignity and intrinsic nobility.

The Sanskrit word for faith is *shraddha*. *Shra-* means heart and *-ddha* is translated to mean place. Therefore, faith is where we place our hearts.[4] If we place our hearts and our attention in the pursuit of the Sleeping World's ideals, our faith is in the machine of Madison Avenue to show us who we are and what is important. If we place our hearts in organic innocence, intrinsic dignity and basic goodness, we will find that our faith is anchored in what is real. Such a faith will give us courage and will sustain us on our journey inward. We will be able to keep digging, going deeper, knowing that we dig to uncover the gold hidden beneath the surface of our awareness, not simply to inventory the garbage pile that may be gathering on top.

Underneath the garbage pile of human pain and suffering is the gold of our true nature, but the process of mining the precious ore of the Self can be arduous and fraught with difficulty. This type of introspective sadhana demands commitment, patience and courage. "Courage," Douglas Brooks tells us, shares the same root (*couer*, in French) as the word "heart." *To have heart* is to have courage. And because as long

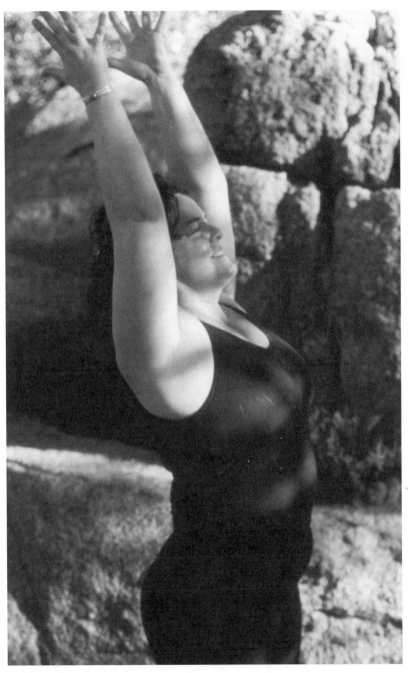

*Urdhva hastasana in tadasana.* Upward facing hands in mountain pose.

as we are alive our heart is beating, we can assume that courage, or having heart, is our most natural state.[5] It is precisely in having heart—in opening our hearts to whatever arises in our lives—that we glimpse our true self and find a pathway to the Divine within.

For those of us who have been at war with the body, the light of the heart is often obscured by the armor of our judgment, obsessions and war-oriented attitudes and behaviors.

*Natrajasana variation.* Dancer pose variation.

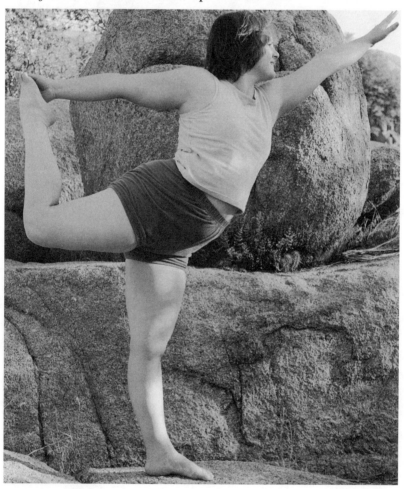

The process of making peace with the body involves taking off the armor that covers our hearts and living more fully in the vulnerability of open-heartedness. Author and spiritual practitioner Regina Sara Ryan writes that opening the heart can be a "dangerous prayer" as it involves opening ourselves to see reality more clearly. And reality can be disturbing.

> Our intention to pray dangerously, which is essentially our willingness to be used for a purpose other than our own comfort and satisfaction, would have the effect of re-enlivening nerve endings long numbed, or melting the walls of ice and snow that we have shored up for protection around our heart. Slowly, inexorably, we start to notice more. We feel more. Transformation is occurring.

> We can't pray, I mean really pray dangerously, unless we have our eyes open to reality. And reality on the planet today is genuinely devastating, heartbreaking. The Buddha said it when he gave us the First Noble Truth: All life is suffering. Not just life in the hospitals. Not just life at the forefront of the war. Not just life in the home where couples are divorcing and using their children as ammunition in their hatred. No, all life. Period . . . No one escapes it. No one.[6]

And so the open heart, our gateway to the Divine, comes with a price tag—we must face reality and reality is suffering. However, the more we open to the reality of suffering, the more we will be able to love and to feel compassion for others. We simply cannot have one without the other. It is through the open heart that we touch suffering and yet is through the same openness that we are touched by the blessings of the Divine. A verse from the *Kularnava Tantra,* an ancient Sanskrit text, states that "By entering the current of the Divine Shakti's descent into heart, the true disciple becomes capable of receiving grace." Douglas Brooks expounds:

> Here in one of the most elegant and subtle statements about yogic practice made anywhere, we are offered a powerful and practical insight: The sincere practitioner of yoga, the true disciple, gains access to the Divine's own creative energy by entering into the Divine's presence which has descended into his or her own heart. By touching the current of Divine grace flowing through our bodies, minds, and hearts, we gain access to an entirely new, awakened and joyous experience of life. What is required of the yogin is to open the heart in order to experience this freely given gift of grace, which naturally flows through our being. To open our hearts to this grace is to experience directly that Divine presence.[7]

Brooks is reminding us that yoga is not an intellectual process—it is a love affair, born in the heart of the true practitioner. We must open our hearts in order to be capable of experiencing grace and to discover our true worth. We are essentially good. We are, by our nature, worthy of receiving grace. In fact, our truest self is ever immersed in the flow of grace. It is only the myth of separation that blinds us to this knowledge and direct experience.

Interestingly, this verse from the *Kularnava Tantra* could also read: "By entering the current of the Divine Shakti's descent into heart, the true disciple becomes *worthy* of receiving grace." In Sanskrit, *worthy* and *capable* are the same word, telling us that essentially there is no distinction between these two states. Therefore our practices are not about proving ourselves *worthy* or even about making us *capable*.[8] The practices are about revealing to us what is essentially true about ourselves in our most natural state, outside of how we feel about ourselves in any moment and untouched by our conditioning and our psychological strategies. Our true worth is not at the mercy of the Sleeping World's demands and expectations. Our original state of essential goodness is not even affected by our behavior. Our spiritual practice allows us to glimpse beyond our false perceptions of ourselves by assisting us to open our hearts to what is true in each moment. The present moment then reveals to us our Divinity where both worthiness and capability come together as one. This is the good news, the great promise.

And still, the payment required of the practitioner is to face suffering with an open heart. It can sound elegant, beautiful and simple to say "we must open the heart." But how does the heart open? I mean truly open wide enough to allow grace to enter in? It breaks open. And in such a way that nothing can relieve the pain of its opening but God. What makes one capable and worthy of receiving grace is a broken heart. I have heard my teacher refer to this broken heart as "a wound that only God can heal." Regina Ryan goes on to tell us that, "only when the heart is truly broken open will we know compassion" for we cannot feel another's pain with a closed heart. And once we truly feel another's pain as our own, the myth of separation begins to crumble.[9] Living with an open heart means that we learn to be with what arises when the heart is no longer protected from the pain that we witness and feel on a daily basis.

## Laura's Story

As far back as I can remember, I had a physical sensation of being very uncomfortable in my own body, as though there was something wrong with it, or it was too big or too heavy. When I was nine, my whole right side was numb for about six months and they really could never find any physiological reason for it. I always had a feeling of not being in my skin. For a long time, if I ate I felt too full and if I didn't eat, I felt too hungry—a constant "dis-ease" in my body. I became bulimic as an attempt to self-medicate; to find a place where it felt okay to be in my skin.

When I walked into class the other day (I have been really feeling fat and dowdy lately and well, depressed) someone told me I looked so svelte. I was immediately aware of how distorted my body image is. I am free and clear of these types of preoccupations for months on end, but it amazing how when anything shifts in my life around relationships, career, finances—that immediately gets registered in my body as a feeling of fat. That is one of the lingering issues or the fall-out of my eating disorder. It is the thing I feel that I can really never get away from. Some people go back to drinking or other behaviors, and me, when I am uncomfortable, I feel fat. When I feel uncomfortable emotionally, it immediately translates into feeling that I am fat.

Yoga has been a central, radiating force behind changes in my relationship to food and my overall health. With yoga there has been a shift from the inside. I find myself making choices about how I eat and how much coffee I drink that are one hundred per-

Making peace with the body means that we do not overeat or restrict calories as a way to numb our hearts or to avoid reality. Practicing peace asks us not to distract ourselves from the bittersweet moments of life with obsessive thoughts about our bodies, our faults and even our perfections—the ways we may measure up to the cultural standard. We stop

cent related to how I want to feel. Through yoga I have been given the ability to feel my body in a way that I like. I like the way my body feels when I eat certain foods. I like the way my body feels when I am done with a very difficult practice or when I wake up and do yoga. My body feels alive, so then I want to feed it so that my body continues to feel alive.

The whole idea that yoga is about progress not perfection is important to me. My whole life has been about posturing and the externals and I don't want yoga to turn into that. It isn't so important how perfectly I do the poses. My goal is not to be able to do the most perfect backbend, but to be able to be brought back into my body every single day. Because I need it. And every single day I need to reaffirm that it is okay to be exactly where I am, since nothing in my background or conditioning has ever told me that. And that is why the community is so important. I can look around and see that we are all connected.

Yoga has been instrumental in my healing. I am learning to be exactly where I am. Instead of feeling preoccupied with my body, I feel tuned into it. Instead of some sort of body dysmorphic pre-occupation, I am now interested in finding a way to tune into my body and its energy and to move it—and that is an incredible gift. My body is stronger than it ever has been. It feels strong, integrated, whole and complete. Being in my body in this new way lends itself to loosening some of the reins about whether I am fat or thin. My life is not just about questioning whether I am fat or thin today. My life is about questioning, do I feel whole?

medicating our pain with daydreams about the future when we "have finally lost our weight," or when our fitness regime has kicked in or when we can achieve a new pose in our yoga practice.

When the heart has been broken in a way that only God can heal then we are ready to receive grace. When we open

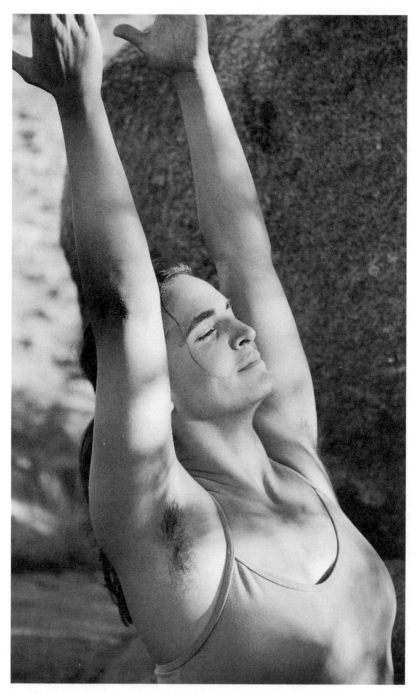

*Urdhva hastasana.* Upward facing hands.

our hearts and when we practice aligning with grace through the practice of hatha yoga, we can allow the tides of self-hatred to turn towards love. We see clearly that the way our body looks is not the source of our pain. We understand that our psychology is not the root source of our suffering. We know that the Sleeping World's answers to these considerations are no longer our answers. We begin to remember our true nature. We begin to see our yoga practice in a new light.

In this new light we can see that on one level the poses we love and practice so faithfully are actually quite incidental. For instance, what if the practice of hatha yoga is simply about uncovering our greatness? Certainly the body will get stronger and more flexible as we learn poses that feel great to practice. However, what if the poses are simply our doorway *in* and a pathway to make offerings back out? As hatha yoga practitioners we can use the poses like Mozart used music, or like a great chef uses food—as a creative medium. The poses can be our tools for exploration and expression, offering us an opportunity for the revelation of grace to occur through them. With our greatness uncovered, we can see the Divine in others and use the asanas as a means to express our innate, natural ecstasy.

Such a spiritual context for asana practice could transform our relationship with our bodies, helping us to create peace and assisting our soul in its evolution. Hatha yoga teaches us to breathe when things are intense, to soften where we are hard and to strengthen where we are weak. It shows us how to bend and how to be steady, how to aspire and how to accept. We learn discipline, commitment, perseverance, how to study and how to teach. Hidden in the forms of the asanas, the alignment technique and breath control is the opportunity to see our true nature and to experience the depth and grandeur of the Divine as it reveals itself in the present moment and through the open heart.

We do not do these practices to earn us freedom or to qualify us for the transmission of grace. We are already present in enlightenment. We are already in a state of grace. We have nothing to earn. We practice simply to uncover, to remember, and to express our essential goodness. In these ways hatha yoga ceases to be an exercise program and becomes instead a spiritual art. Practicing hatha yoga as a spiritual art is teaching me how to make peace with my body, how to open my heart more fully and in so doing, how to avail myself to the flow of grace.

# CHAPTER SIX

# *Accepting "What Is"*

For me to remain open to my teacher's influence, or for any of us to offer ourselves to the Divine, is to surrender to the way things are. That means accepting our husband or wife as he or she is, our students as they are, our parents as they are, our coworkers as they are, the weather as it is and our body as it is. Through self-observation and paying attention we hone our ability to see more accurately. Through our intention to make peace and our willingness to align our actions with our intention, we practice the art of accepting the body as it is. The art of self-acceptance is not a mysterious practice that we suddenly find ourselves able to do. We begin exactly where we are, often in the small details of our daily routines and mundane behaviors.

My sister once told me a story that pointed out how much I don't want to accept what is. She was attending a yoga intensive with a masterful yogini from India who remarked to the group that yoga teachers should never wear black tights because it is impossible for their students to see what their legs really looked like in black tights.

When I heard this statement, I thought, "That is exactly *why* I wear black tights—to hide what my legs really look like!" I remembered the countless internalized instructions about dressing to hide "figure flaws," such as: always wear black to slim down the appearance of heavy hips and thighs, or never wear horizontal stripes. In the Sleeping World we are encouraged to hide what doesn't meet the cultural standard of perfection, even when the standard is completely unrealistic, and even though the fat or any other perceived flaw is still present, whether or not it can be seen. We douse ourselves in deodorants and perfumes, and squeeze ourselves into "figure enhancing" undergarments. We color our hair when it turns gray and bleach our teeth when they are no longer sparkly white. The examples of this phenomenon are endless. We continually hide "what is" from each other and from ourselves. We mask the reality of our body as it is and attempt to appear differently than we are.

In a context of yoga and awakening, the master teacher says, "We must *see* what is happening in the legs." She certainly is not referring to seeing the things we try to hide with black tights—stretch marks, cellulite, size, girth, freckles, dimples, varicose veins, pale skin or body hair. She is not concerned about the initial appearance of the body according to the standards of the Sleeping World. She wants students to be able to see the deeper truth of correct alignment and muscular action—the reality of the hatha yogi.

I took this teacher's advice. I began wearing shorts designed for yoga—I call them my "bloomers." They are short and slightly baggy, with elasticized leg bands, and are certainly not flattering by any conventional standard. However, they have offered fuel for my sadhana. First, they provide much greater freedom of movement. I find the bloomers infinitely more natural feeling and comfortable than Spandex or Lycra tights. I am more able to access the muscles of my buttocks and legs. The bloomers do not bind, pinch or suck me in, in an attempt to make me appear smaller than I am. Without the tightness of Spandex I can use my leg muscles with more precision and sensitivity. Metaphorically, more freedom, less constriction and greater sensitivity are a constant reminding factor of some of the possible fruits of sadhana and spiritual life.

Secondly, the shorts hide very little physically. My entire leg can be seen. The stretch marks on my legs are there for all to see. They speak of the many times when, due to my internal struggles, I over-ate and gained weight. My cellulite is on display. So is the fact that I am not tanned. All of the things that are true beneath black tights are also true in bloomers. However, when I am wearing the shorts, the truth is not hidden. In this small practice of allowing my body to be seen as it is, I do not engage the game of the Sleeping World.

When I first began wearing these bloomers I would find my insecurity surfacing. "You are the yoga teacher, you are supposed to look fit and thin," my mind would lament. I found I could answer back, "I am the yoga teacher and a yoga practitioner, I am supposed to *be* authentic. This is what is real about my body today, what is real about me. I have short legs with some fat on them and no tan. Is that so wrong? Does that diminish any expertise I have to offer a group of students? Does that diminish the value of my practice?"

Through this process I aligned another piece of my behavior with my intention to make peace. As simple as it may sound, the small act of altering what I wore to practice yoga shifted my relationship with my body. Making peace is not an intellectual process. Making peace happens by continually confronting my beliefs and taking small steps that align with an intention greater than my conditioning. To say that I

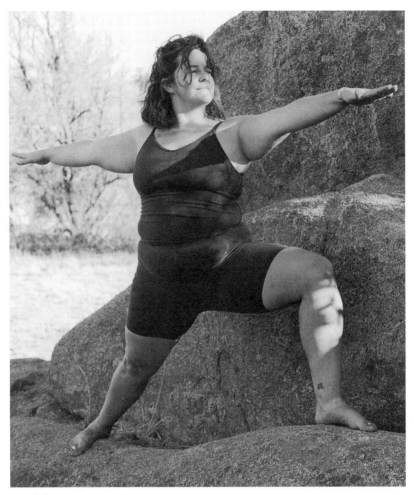

*Virabhadrasana II.* Warrior pose variation 2.

want to make peace but to continue to hide from *what is* real, is counter-productive. Accepting what is is keeping the covenant of peace.

The practice of being with ourselves, as we are in the moment, is a fundamental practice of many spiritual traditions. French spiritual teacher Arnaud Desjardins implores us to practice saying "yes" to life, telling us that "the fundamental practice is always here and now: to convert the refusal into acceptance."[1] Whatever it is that we are refusing holds us hostage and demands our energy to keep it in the darkness of denial. Once allowed into the light of acceptance, the very thing we have refused has a chance to be transformed.

> The only way that you can open up is through the most magical word of all, the supreme mantra . . .yes. "Yes" is the translation of *aum:* the letter A—"yes" to Brahma, the letter "U" —"yes" to Vishnu, the letter "M" —"yes" to Shiva. Listening is the ear's "yes" ; looking is the eye's "yes" ; smelling is the nose's "yes" ; tasting is the "yes" of the tongue and the palate; touching is the "yes" of sensation. The only way you can open up is through "yes." Someone knocks at the door, you decide to welcome him, you say, "Come in" or "Yes." Refusing to open up is the same thing as saying "No."

> You have been taught not to say "yes" to the life force, to spontaneity, movement, joy, expansion: "No, you won't express yourself, no you won't grow up, no you won't be fulfilled!" And you have ended up making this "no" a part of yourself. Nonetheless, life remains intact and "yes" is the oath leading back to it. It is a magic word. Both are magic words, "no" just as much as "yes" (but one will destroy you and the other will save you.)[2]

Saying "yes" we create peace with the body and experience our true nature without apology, shame or recoil. In this same spirit, Desjardins' own Indian spiritual teacher, Swami Prajnanpad, advised his devotees to *welcome* whatever it is that life was offering them in the present moment. "Welcome to this perception, welcome to that sensation, welcome to what is new, welcome to what disturbs me."[3] When we welcome whatever is arising internally and externally we are living in the moment. In the act of accepting ourselves as we are, and life as it is in the moment, we are actually living in the flow of grace. John Friend outlines the same sentiment beautifully in describing the essence of *anusara,* a Sanskrit word that means to "flow with grace":

> Anusara is flowing with Grace, saying yes! to the whole spectrum of the magic of life. It is a willingness to be aware of all parts of ourselves—the light and the dark, the full rainbow of sensation, perception, emotion and thought. To be in the flow is to look at whatever arises with freshness and freedom. It is simply to open our hearts with love to the present moment without clinging or pushing. Anusara is accepting the world and ourselves as we are, and then responding with love.[4]

Yoga teacher and practitioner, Sam Dworkis, suggests that:

Enhanced flexibility, strength, and endurance need not be yoga's goal. The "goal" needs to be to learn how to pay attention to "what is." "What is" is how you feel right now. "What is" is not *trying* to get your hands to the floor; or *trying* to do a headstand or *trying* to do a back bend, or *trying* to do any particular yoga exercise. Most importantly, an appropriate yoga practice is not *trying* to get your body to feel like it may have felt in the past or *trying* to get your body to feel like you think it should feel. If you were supposed to be different, you would already be there. An appropriate yoga practice, therefore, is not about *trying;* it is about non-aggressively doing . . . it is about *being.*[5]

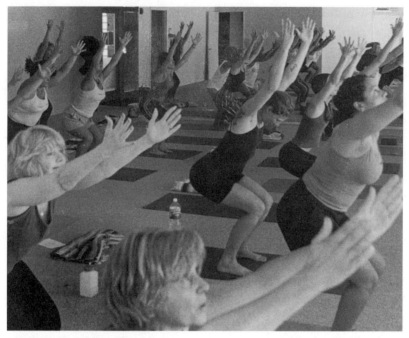

*Urdhva hastasana in tadasana.* Upward facing hands in mountain pose.

Allowing ourselves to be in the moment, non-aggressively doing what is wanted and needed is a spiritual practice. In so many ways we are conditioned to run away from the present moment in search of some relief in the future or some comforting reverie of the past.

## Gratitude for What Is

Life as it is, in the moment, is a gift from the Divine—"the present." How many times a day do we refuse the gift by complaining, avoiding, or compulsively attempting to bend reality to our whim rather than simply surrendering to the way that things are? We think nothing of exchanging something we have been given for something we perceive as better. (God forbid we actually wear a shirt we didn't like very much as a way to honor the gift giver.) When our body doesn't meet our expectations we criticize it, dress in ways that hide it and try to manipulate our appearance through diets and exercise. We even custom order body parts from plastic surgeons rather than face our feelings of inferiority and insecurity with how we are in the moment.

When we step away from this consumer mentality and enter into spiritual life we practice seeing the present moment as a gift—perfectly designed for us to learn from. We remember that if we were supposed to be different in this very moment, we would be. If life were supposed to be different right now, it would be. We use our yoga practice to observe ourselves as we are, rather than for how we aren't good enough. When we accept our life as it is and our body as it is and when our yoga practice reflects this type of acceptance, we are making peace. Metaphorically, we are aligning ourselves with the ancient ritual of exchanging *prasad.*

Prasad, a Sanskrit word meaning "grace," is literally the food that has been offered to a deity, which is then shared among devotees as God's gift and blessing.[6] The ritual offering of prasad takes place when the devotee presents a gift to the master and receives a gift in return. When we offer our practice and ourselves to the Divine as prasad, we get back the gift of the present moment. When we fail to accept the present moment, just as it is, we are refusing the gift the Divine has given us. We are refusing to participate in the exchange of prasad. Imagine the Divine Itself giving you a present and you saying, "Well, thank you but I would really prefer it in a different size and color. Perhaps I could just exchange it—you won't mind, will you?" When we accept our bodies and our lives in the present moment just as they are, we complete the ritual exchange

## Deborah's Story

*Deborah, my yoga student, is diabetic and overweight. Her extra weight is a real health concern. After attempting to lose weight through force and imposed violent extremes, she is finding that the only way to affect lasting change in her physical body is to engage in a practice of acceptance and making peace. Hatha yoga has been integral to her peacemaking process.*

Years ago I had lost a whole lot of weight, maybe sixty pounds. And the way I did it was from a very materialistic point of view. Because I had never lifted weights before and I had never been athletic, I just fell into all of the pitfalls that people who work out compulsively fall into. Instead of it making me more vulnerable and more available to my husband and my friends, it actually armored me, even though I lost all of this weight and I looked better.

Slowly, tragically, heartbreakingly, the weight came back on and then with a combination of rigorous exercise and not being sensitive to my body, I wound up with tendinitis in my ankles and I couldn't do anything for a long time, not even walk.

About a year ago I started to take yoga classes because it was the only thing I could think of that my body could do. Everybody else in the class was like seventy years old and the class was so basic and so elementary. But I didn't care. I was so relieved and

of prasad. Acceptance is the way we open the gift we have been given, use it to its fullest potential and say "thank you."

Acceptance should not be used to justify patterns of thinking and behaving that are outdated and that may be causing harm. However, lasting change comes from an unconditional acceptance of the place in which we are, in the moment. For instance, if we are planning a road trip from California to New York, the road maps will only be useful if

happy to be moving my body again and for someone to direct me in how to move in a way that was healthy for me.

Doing the yoga has been a foundation for getting me back into doing other forms of exercise, like aerobic exercise and some weightlifting, but from a totally different perspective. I am exercising so I can be healthy. It's not about vanity. It isn't about looking in the mirror. I don't want to be a diabetic who has to take insulin in five years. I want my blood pressure to go down. I am happy with my life and I want to keep living it instead of dying.

Now it is really time. If I am going to be able to live long enough to be able to give back to my life, to the people around me and to everything around me that is important to me, I have to take care of my body. It is a matter of life and death. It is making the decision to live.[7]

*Deborah's decision to keep living came in part from an honest appraisal of the ways in which she was dying. Her decision to make peace with her body came from an honest evaluation of the war that she had waged for most of her life. And although her issues are far from resolved, Deborah has made a certain peace with the way she approaches her process. She describes herself as a "muddler" and although her practice of making peace with herself has been slow and laborious she has been practicing accepting herself "as someone who may just muddle through this for quite some time."[8]*

we honestly acknowledge that our starting point is California. If we pretend we are in Vermont and then plan our trip according to those road maps, we will get lost. Signs along the way will have no meaning, directions we ask for will seem to lead us astray and we will not know where the next place is to rest or refuel. We must fully accept our starting point to successfully navigate the journey we want to make. If we say we want to make peace with the body and then fail to acknowledge the seriousness of the war in which we are engaged, our efforts will be thwarted from the outset. Sometimes an honest appraisal of the way things are shows us that it is appropriate to take action toward changing our bodies. But taking action toward change does not mean that we do not accept ourselves in the moment.

## The Heart of the Matter

Whatever our particular process of making peace with the body looks like, we can be sure that we will be asked to accept ourselves as we are before we will be able to make any lasting changes in our outlook and in our behavior. When I

*Eka pada rajakapotasana I.* One leg royal king pigeon pose, variation 1.

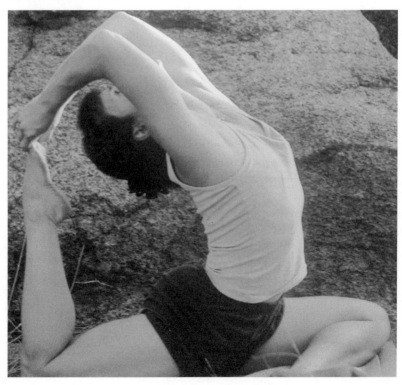

asked my teacher, Lee, what he thought was a healthy relationship with the body he said, "Well, first of all would be acceptance of the body exactly as it is."[9] John Friend responded similarly saying,

> One of the components of healthy body image would be to have a clear realistic perception of oneself. Let's say that whether you are skinny or overweight, you wouldn't try to say, "I am really fine." You can say, "I am really thin" or "I'm really big" and you can still find the good in what the reality is. So the first thing is acceptance about what really is. And that's not easy because even when you think you really see yourself, you probably don't. But as best as we can, we try to see ourselves clearly and accept that.
>
> Then finding the good in it and then really knowing and taking the premise that every person and all of the diversity that people can exhibit, there is a purpose and a reason. Like in a garden. You want a whole variety of flowers to really make it beautiful . . . And each is not like the other. And the whole diversification represents the freedom of the Supreme to manifest in that particular form.
>
> Also another thing that goes along with body image is the intention to manifest oneself as beautifully and as healthily as possible. I think it would be hypocritical for someone who was not exercising or eating properly to say, "Oh, I am fine." That is not a healthy body image to me. That is a false healthy body image. But let's say you are eating well and you are exercising and you are still kind of big or even overweight

and you just say, "I am doing the best I can." That is a healthy body image. You try to align yourself and be as healthy as possible. You do the best you can and then you let it go because that is just the way it is. That is just the way you are.[10]

Ironically, change will often happen once we accept ourselves or the situation that we find intolerable. However, we must first accept reality fully. Many times we will try to pretend that we have accepted something, saying to ourselves, "If I accept this situation then it will change." But there really is no shortcut in the work of acceptance. Acceptance means that we have made such peace with a situation that we are ready to live with it as it is forever, as though it may never change. We may *never* lose weight, we may *never* balance in a headstand, we may *never* sit in lotus pose, our partner may *never* wash their dishes in a timely manner, our child may *never* get straight A's. Sometimes if we are having difficulty accepting an aspect of reality the best we can do is accept ourselves in our non-acceptance. Accepting ourselves exactly as we are in the moment is one of the most loving things we can do for ourselves. And self-love is one of the most crucial aspects of making peace with the body. John Friend continues:

At the heart of all this self-acceptance is self-love and self-appreciation. When we turn love back on ourselves like that, I can't think of anything more healing and transformative spiritually. For me, it might be at the root of all spiritual work—self-honoring and self-love . . . When you just accept like that, a new opening happens. Your ability to open to other people to see beauty in everything. Life just starts to seem brighter.[11]

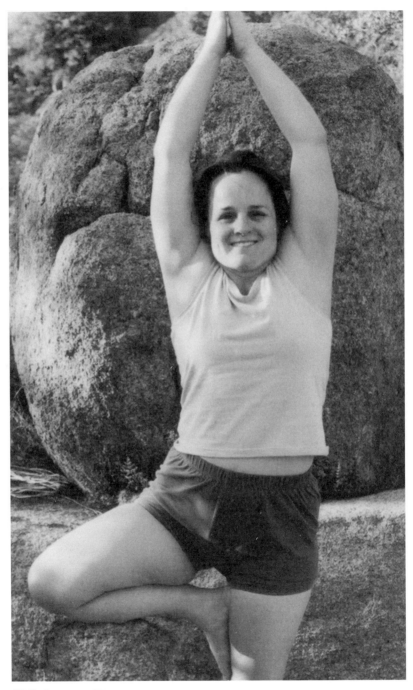

*Vrikshasana.* Tree pose.

In the brightness of openhearted acceptance we begin to experience the practice of alignment in hatha yoga as a means for self-observation as well as a means for self-honoring. As we learn to pay attention to the alignment of the body, the mind and the spirit, we learn to accept ourselves as we are, our bodies as they are and our life as it is. It is through the ongoing practice of honoring "what is" in its many manifestations, that we infuse our yoga with objectivity, honest feedback, and offerings of peace and love.

# CHAPTER SEVEN

# Hatha Yoga as a Spiritual Art

*A pose can have exquisite alignment and be balanced in its Action, but without a pure spiritual expression from the heart, it loses its power for deep inner transformation. A pure spiritual expression in a posture is an unfolding of the deepest qualities of the heart, such as love and joy, into the body and surrounding environment. These pure heart qualities make a posture sing with a beautiful inner music, which harmoniously joins into the grand symphony of life. This heart energy (pure attitude) is the key element that makes the practice of hatha yoga into a profoundly transformational art. A pure attitude during the performance of an asana purifies the body and mind, and lets the light of the heart freely shine out.*

—John Friend

Yoga magazines and advertisements for yoga products and workshops—in short, the *industry* of yoga—sell images of beauty identical to those of the Sleeping World. Women are pictured as thin, blemish-free examples of health and spiritual evolution. Men are strong, muscular, lean and good-looking by cultural definitions. Yoga today is continually sold with the same promises as are aerobics classes and workout videos—weight loss, thinner thighs, flatter abdominals and tighter buns. Even loftier promises such as peace of mind, relaxation, and expanded awareness are often packaged for profit. One ad for a yoga teacher-training course actually lures the prospective teacher to this particular program with the slogan "Learn to set souls free." Another popular studio advertises their method and classes saying, "Get a Bikram‡ butt."

When we allow our sadhana, our spiritual practice, to be motivated by the Sleeping World's commercialization of yoga, we are participating in the war against ourselves through the practice of yoga. When we attend yoga classes where there is a primary emphasis on toning, shaping, losing weight, criticizing or changing the body's appearance rather than on accepting the body as it is, we are at war. When we practice yoga and indulge in self-talk that is negative, discouraging, comparative and judgmental, then we have broken the treaty of peace. To practice hatha yoga as a peace offering we learn to practice this ancient art and science in a way that is objective and free of the cultural influences that have created the war with the body in the first place.

An "objective practice is a practice that holds the possibility of literal transformation within its form. The form of an objective practice is empowered and therefore can transmit/communicate the truth, the real, the universal."[1] Examples of objective practice include many methods of meditation, mantra repetition, ritual dance, and certain types of sacred art such as sand mandalas or thangka painting. Georg Feuerstein, one of the most highly regarded yoga scholars in the West, points to hatha yoga's potential as an objective practice stating that, "Hatha Yoga was originally conceived as a full liberation technology and may still be practiced as such."[2]

‡Bikram refers to Bikram Choudhury, who developed a very athletic form of yoga.

The original context for the practice of hatha yoga was the transformation of the human being from ego-centered to God-centered. "In its most archaic form, Yoga was a combination of ritual worship and meditation, having the purpose of opening the gates to the celestial realms and beyond."[3] "The word 'yoga' originates from the Sanskrit root *yuj* which means Union. On the spiritual plane, it means union of the Individual Self with the Universal Self; while for the man of this world, it is the union of the physical, physiological, mental, emotional and intellectual bodies leading one to live an integrated purposeful, useful and noble life."[4]

Depending upon the intention of the practitioner, hatha yoga can be a devotional offering to the self and to the Divine, or it can be yet another way for the separative ego to reinforce the myth of its existence and of its importance. For hatha yoga to have ultimate meaning we must become serious practitioners. We must examine whether we are interested in simply posing or in truly practicing, and true practice begins with intention.

Certainly all of the trends within the popularization of yoga are not bad or wrong. Yoga is often taught in health clubs, or in seminars in which yogic methodology is applied to help people manage stress or to cope with back pain, for instance. I am not criticizing people who practice or teach yoga simply as another method of keeping the body healthy. Yoga as a physical regime has benefited many. Making the body stronger and more resilient allows many people to feel better emotionally as well as physically. I have several students whose primary reason for practicing yoga is rooted in maintaining the physical health of their bodies, and these students have very little interest in yoga philosophy, chant-

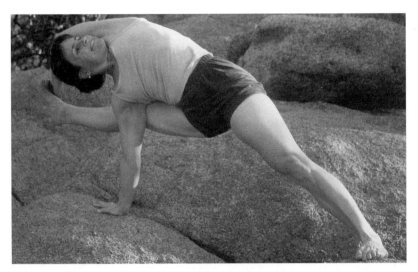

*Vishvamitrasana.* Vishvamitra's pose. Vishvamitra was a sage.

ing, meditation or anything overtly spiritual. They will likely not engage a relationship with a guru or spiritual teacher. They still love practicing yoga and they enjoy great benefit from the asanas and from the community of practitioners.

I am grateful that hatha yoga is readily available and I personally have benefited from its increasing popularity. Many people who never would have sought out hatha yoga in an ashram, for instance, have been brought to serious practice and study because of the accessibility of "modern yoga." I am happy we have yoga props, supplies, books, magazines and accouterments galore, readily available to us to assist us in our practice. What is important here, however, is to remember that hatha yoga is at its roots, a spiritual practice, not a competition, a fashion show, a merchandising opportunity or a popularity contest. The more trappings, glamour and "stuff" that we, as a culture of practitioners, surround hatha yoga with, the more we risk losing sight of the true purpose of the practice.

However, when hatha yoga is a means to making peace with our bodies and to transforming the context of our lives, we must begin to look deeper into the possibility that the practice offers us. We must begin to embrace the totality of what the practice of hatha yoga is. The war we have learned to perpetuate against our bodies and ourselves is a spiritual problem. Our vanities, our insecurity, our obsession with perfection, the prevalence of obesity, the increase of eating disorders and stress-related illnesses—all of these are manifestations of our perceived spiritual emptiness, our spiritually bereft culture, and our attachment to the ideals of the Sleeping World. Since it is a spiritual dilemma about which we are talking, the solution is also *spiritual*. Practicing yoga without honoring its spiritual roots and aligning with its true context simply won't get the same job done.

## Surrender versus Perfection

*When you have a construction business, you need people who can work—but God can succeed with people who are twisted and lost. That's the genius of God!*
—Arnaud Desjardins

One day after several stressful months of work at the coffee shop that my husband and I own and operate, I found myself at the point of exasperation and close to tears. I called a senior practitioner from my spiritual community for support. She listened patiently as I cried about how poorly I was managing my stress, how rude I had been to the customers, how terrible I was at being a boss, and basically what a spiritual loser I was. When I finally came up for air, she said, "You know, we often forget that spiritual work is not about getting perfect—this work is about being surrendered."

I was quite shocked. I don't think my rational mind even believed her but my heart did. I began to reflect on how through all my years of therapy, therapy training, and yoga practice I was striving to be perfect so that I would be lovable. I imagined that if I did enough work on myself I would no longer have neurotic manifestations or offensive personality traits. She was telling me that such an idealized state wasn't even the point. Surrender was the point, if there is a point at all to the crazy wisdom of the Divine.

My friend went on to suggest that I find some way to practice compassion for myself and to simply start over. She suggested that I try to let go of my self-condemnation for my recent behavior and begin a new moment. She suggested I soften towards myself. She reminded me that self-observation is not intended to be used as a weapon against myself.

Since that conversation, I have often heard my spiritual teacher speak about how *trying* to rid ourselves of all of our quirks and personality traits is actually a waste of valuable work energy. He suggests that we simply manage our personality so that it doesn't significantly affect our ability to have relationships and meaningful work—to be involved in daily life. Freud, too, said that the goal of psychotherapy was for the patient to be able to love and work. He did not designate psychological perfection as the successful outcome of psychotherapy.[5]

The ability to love and work might also be the successful outcome of spiritual practice. To love would mean to surrender to the guru or to the Divine; to devote oneself to God in such a way that our psychological fears do not hinder our heart's calling to our true path. Such love would be full in the direct experience of the present moment, just as it is. To work

## Anne-Marie's Story

*Having studied philosophy and comparative religion, Anne-Marie's initial interest in yoga was for stress reduction and as a break from these intellectual pursuits. Through the kaya sadhana of hatha yoga not only did the intellectual, spiritual and physical meet, but a long history of struggle with the body began to resolve and transform.*

From an early age, like 9 or 10, I got the strong message that I was too heavy and that I needed to drink diet soda and eat less. I don't think I was objectively fat, but I lived as if I was; or that being fat was always lurking just around the corner. Since I really loved food, I felt mad at my body for not letting me eat whatever I wanted. As I got older I definitely internalized all the familial and societal messages to be thin and I self-policed pretty excessively. I developed eating disorders, and all that. At some points I was objectively slender, but I never really experienced myself as a thin person and I didn't experience a sense of satisfaction with my body. It was never quite right. Also I was active in sports but I never excelled at them so I had this feeling that my body wasn't strong enough, or fast enough.

would be to surrender to the sometimes-excruciating demands of practice, selfless service, and the relief of suffering without concern that our own needs weren't being met. In many ways, to love and work would mean not having our *own* life but instead for God to have our life. In order to love and work in these ways we must surrender ourselves, not perfect ourselves.

When I bring this consideration of surrender rather than perfection to my yoga practice, I am aligning myself with my intention to make peace. On the other hand, the practice of hatha yoga can be fertile ground in which to sow the seeds of perfectionism and constant dissatisfaction. The refining

Yoga has definitely made me focus on my body in terms of what it can do and less in terms of what it can't do. I think yoga also made me calmer and more spiritual, and that has allowed me to be less anxious and gripped around more superficial issues. It has also helped me overcome certain feelings of fear or unwillingness to look at the body very deeply. The demand for attention to the present moment in hatha yoga, meditation and pranayama (breathing exercises) practice and also the focus on precision and alignment hooked me on an intellectual level and so I started looking at the body more objectively.

Sometimes I wish I was making faster progress toward padmasana, (lotus pose) but yoga lets me see that for what it is too, just competitiveness or lack of self-acceptance. I just do what I can do and be here now.

By looking at other people's bodies in yogic terms I see the thin or the muscle-bound body as limited or unnatural looking. Seeing lots of different bodies all trying to do the same pose is useful and humbling. Also, seeing how other people deal with body issues—fears and anxieties that come up in class—has made me feel less alone in the dislike of the body. My teacher's studio has none of the "yoga-for-weight-loss" energy, so it is a kind of safe haven.

of the asanas is endless, much like the refinement possible in other areas of sadhana. Yoga masters tell us that they are able to move their muscles in one way and their skin in another. They can control the movement of their hair follicles. Their respiration is under their control and many can stop and start the beating of their heart.

Truly there is no end to practice. Even if we learn how to choose our last breath, once the physical body is gone we are simply transported to the next stage of learning and practice. Perfection isn't even possible. What a relief to know that perfection isn't the goal.

Fourth Way teacher E.J. Gold says that, at the end of our lives, when we are on our deathbeds, we will not be remembering the myriad of things that so occupy our minds today—the details and dramas of our existence. Instead we will be called to consider how well we have loved:

> Lying there in our deathbeds, we finally understand that the only thing left is our breath, God's love for us and our love for God and anything we might have done to really work on and with the essential part of ourselves. All of the pressing urgencies and ambitions of life are now seen for what they really are—worthless . . . [death] has a certain atmosphere of reality to it . . . it brings you to a point where you suddenly recognize your values in life, what's really, really important to you.[6]

When we are dying I don't think we will be reflecting on the appearance of our body according to Sleeping World standards, or the perfection of our asanas or anything else. At that point I hope I do not care about how many stunning backbends I did or how thin I finally got my body to be. Instead, I hope my yoga practice will have cultivated qualities of discrimination, introspection, open-heartedness, courage, commitment and dedication that will allow me a greater ability to love. I hope that when I reflect on my life I am able to see that such qualities have born the fruit of loving relationships and useful service. I hope that by the very act of accepting myself as I am and my body as it is when I practice yoga—in other words, the very process of making peace with myself, of practicing from the inside out—I will have forged a different kind of body, a body of work, through which I will have served the Divine.

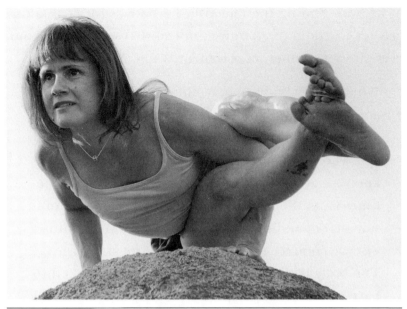

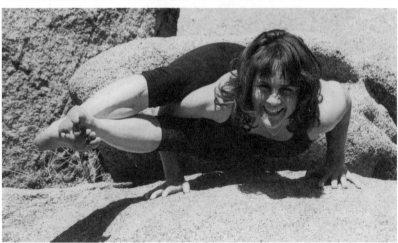

*Astavakrasana.* Astavakra's pose. Astavakra was a sage.

The "body of work" will last past the point of our physical death and so ultimately it is much more important to our spiritual growth than the physical body. We must remember that as vital as peace with the body may be to our personal growth, the process should not become an obsession or a compulsion

111

of its own. Ending the war with the body is for facilitating greater freedom of attention, not so that we consume our lives with yet another set of standards and methods.

> What is your body anyway but a bag of shit and pus and mucus? You'll find out, some of you, when you're 80 years old, what your body is really made of. Any of you who have been around people who are dying know . . . it's mortality in spades. And it rots. Sometimes from the inside out, sometimes from the outside in, depending on what kind of rot you contract —if you contract a particular form of rot as you age . . . The body is only the body. And you really need to have a little bit of perspective; it's only the body and it will go some day.[7] —*Lee Lozowick*

While this message isn't delivered in gentle terms, it is a potent reminder that we are involved in a process of making peace with the body so that we can move our attention from ego-centered self-hatred to God-centered service and devotion. Although the physical body will certainly go one day, Lee Lozowick has said that after the physical "body is dead, your subtle bodies are still going to be alive and kicking. So really in the process of your sadhana, you need to be paying at least as much attention to the nutrition your subtle bodies are getting over and against the nutrition that this gross body gets."[8]

The practice of hatha yoga with proper intention affords us an excellent opportunity to feed the subtle body as we care for and use the physical form in our sadhana. In fact, this entire book has been about cultivating a practice of hatha yoga that feeds us the "food" of compassion and peace rather than the junk food of the Sleeping World's standards for our physical structure. A steady diet of respect, acceptance, and honest self-observation is called for in the process of creating a new relationship with the body. Hatha yoga, good company, the guru or teacher, and self-observation are the soul food that nourish and sustain us on many levels.

## The Guru

*How do we distinguish between the true guru and the false one? The cult of the guru, or master, is an Asian concept. To other societies, the concept might seem exotic, mysterious, or even abhorrent, a brake on individual freedom or judgment. Some thinkers have declared that a guru is not needed at all, while others believe that you cannot reach your goal without one. Perhaps the importance of the guru can be explained by examining its Sanskrit root. Gu means "darkness" and* ru *means "light." Therefore, a guru is one who leads you from darkness to light.*
—B.K.S. Iyengar

Recently I spoke to a friend about my book. She asked me if I was going to mention the fact that I had a spiritual teacher. "Of course," I said, "not because it is the easiest subject to write about, but because every bit of progress I have made with these issues has happened since I have come into my teacher's company. Being with him has radically changed my relationship with my body and my practice of hatha yoga. To write about the subject without mentioning my teacher—my guru—just wouldn't be honest." Simply put, hatha yoga is a way for me to access my guru and to practice his teachings in a tangible, dynamic form.

Much has been published on the guru-disciple relationship over the years. Volumes exist about the abuses of power, the deceptions and the reasons why we do not need to submit ourselves to the will of a guru. Equally extensive are the stories of the ecstasies, the triumphs over ego that have been attained by keeping the company of saints, and the arguments about why the guru is absolutely necessary in order to evolve spiritually.

People in either camp are certainly not looking to be convinced in a direction other than their position and so this debate is usually quite pointless. In my opinion, much of the popular rhetoric about the necessity of the guru misses one crucial point. My experience of working with a guru is that the relationship is not one that is decided based on logic or

*Parivritta prasarita padottanasana.* Revolved wide stance forward bend.

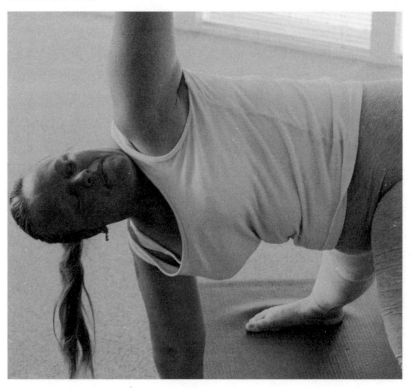

on a prescribed set of spiritual rules. The decision to work with a guru is a decision of the heart, not the intellect. The question is not whether the guru is necessary but rather, *if* we are being called to be with a guru, how can we best surrender ourselves to that calling?

The relationship with the guru is one that is made outside of time and space. In my case, I believe that the decision to study with my spiritual teacher was made before I was "Christina" and before my guru was "Lee Lozowick." Deciding to be in relationship with Lee was about aligning with a decision that had already been made, and a truth that was already established. Certainly I had intellectual reservations that surfaced during my approach to him and to his community. However, what I found was that the decision to work with my teacher was already made in my heart and the intellectual arguments fell away with little fanfare.

It is certainly okay to live without a guru. A vast number of honest, loving, compassionate people with great integrity who do great work have never consciously aligned themselves with a guru. One can grow and mature and serve others and not have a guru.

In the same way, it is okay to *have* a guru. For those of us who do, the guru is absolutely necessary. For us, attempting spiritual life without the guru would be like trying to breathe without lungs. Why would we not want to have the assistance, the Divine love, and the constant blessing force that comes through a human guru? Even the irritation that the guru can provide is something that we can learn to treasure. We believe that the undoing of the personal self is necessary in order to shift the context of our lives from self-centered to God-centered. We assume that the ego will never be able to truly see to its own undoing, even though the ego certainly does an excellent job of convincing us that it can undo itself.

Georg Feuerstein echoes this sentiment,

> To practice Tantra Yoga without the initiatory grace of an adept amounts to a Sisyphean task; uninitiated seekers are engaged in pushing the massive boulder of their own karma uphill, and what awaits them in the end is either discouragement or self-delusion. Only the graceful intervention of an adept both lessens the weight of the karmic boulder and infuses the practitioner's muscles with the necessary strength to reach the top of the mountain of inner growth. Because spiritual initiation is not a concept in our modern Western Culture, however, few people can appreciate the unique opportunity this represents. Instead they worry about issues of power and exploitation. Their concerns have been fueled in recent years by exposés in the news media about the irresponsible and even abusive behavior of several well-known spiritual teachers. But these frailties say nothing about the tradition of initiation itself, which is as potent and relevant as ever.[9]

Feuerstein goes on to compare the guru tradition to mathematics, saying that mathematics "is a perfectly valid symbol system. But there are good and not-so-good math teachers, who either succeed or fail (sometimes completely) to communicate that system and its intrinsic intellectual beauty to their pupils."[10] And so it is with gurus. There are plenty of spiritual teachers from many different traditions who have misused their power and who have caused pain and suffering to the people in whom they inspired trust. And there are spiritual teachers who help their devotees to lighten their suffering and who can consistently communicate the intrinsic beauty of the Divine to their students.

Ultimately the guru is not a person—the guru is a function or a principle. It is this function that allows the Divine to become accessible to the individual. "The Guru serves as the tangent point between the human domain and the Divine . . . without this tangent point, the two do not meet."[11] In this way, the guru serves as a sort of mediator for the disciple, helping the disciple to consciously align to Divine intelligence. The guru function serves to destroy our illusions and to assist us in waking up from the Sleeping World's egoic dream. "The 'guru function' primarily consists in constantly and faithfully mirroring the disciples back to themselves, while at the same time strengthening their intuition of the ultimate reality, the transcendental self. Because of this dual aspect, the guru's work with disciples is both a demolition job and a rebuilding."[12]

Jesus Christ performed this guru function for his disciples. In ancient Greece, Socrates and other great teachers performed the guru function for their students. Traditionally, hatha yoga instruction was transmitted through this guru function.

With the industrialization of yoga, we now receive yogic teachings in health clubs, fancy yoga studios, recreation centers and through videos, magazines, television infomercials, popular books and CDs. As hatha yoga is so often packaged as simply another health-related regime, the original context for the practice is often lost and its relationship to the guru function is obscured from sight so as not to make Western yoga consumers uncomfortable with hatha yoga's spiritual roots. While the sacred function of teaching hatha yoga now rests in the media's hands, the public grows ever more cynical and fearful of genuine spiritual masters and adherence to tradition. Students skip from instructor to instructor, from method to method, never feeling the need to commit to a tradition or a style, and therefore miss the benefits that focused study and a long term, in-depth relationship with one teacher can provide. Yoga teachers often teach a "synthesis" of styles that is nothing more than a conglomeration of things that they are good at, comfortable with, and that they find profitable. I have been at teacher training seminars where teachers said they don't teach detailed alignment because "the students find that stopping to study the poses in depth interferes with the flow of their workout." These teachers have allowed the people they teach to become customers rather than students.

The guru functions as a source of energy and the devotee must learn to plug him or herself into the power source in order to take advantage of what is being offered. For me, hatha yoga is one of the ways I "plug in."

My yoga teacher, John Friend, is a devotee of Gurumayi Chidvilasanada. He told me once that he believes that the relationship with the guru is something one can only understand from having a personal experience of it. I asked him how his relationship with Gurumayi affected his hatha yoga practice. He replied:

When I felt Her Presence, I felt a real, tangible presence that was apparently emanating from her but was moving within me and it was able to make great shifts

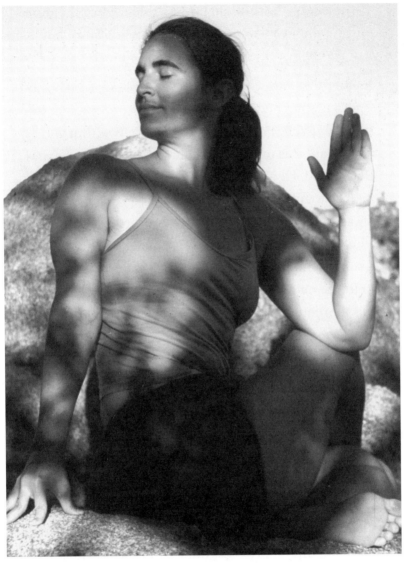

*Ardha matsyendrasana.* Matsyendra's pose. Matsyendra was a sage.

within my body, mind and spirit. Then I learned to soften and attune to that energy more, instead of hardening. What I used to do is just try to do it by myself, so I ended up just being harder. But when I tuned to the energy by softening, I was able to do a lot more and it came from not only being more sensitive but by respecting myself more and having self-love.

So, her first and foremost, her most paramount teaching to me has always been, "Meditate on yourself. Respect yourself. For God lives and dwells within you as you." I am this uniqueness that they call John . . . and that is God. He's chosen to take that form and I should be respectful to that. And that shifted everything. Then I was starting to be sweet to myself instead of being tough to myself and then sweet to everyone else. And that just shifted my practice. The way that I bent and held myself and breathed and twisted and everything was more in relationship with that Self.

She guided me like that. She was strong enough—her energy was strong enough—that I literally felt it inside. It was something! I never felt like that before . . . It was really Real.[13]

John's experience of the guru's influence describes very clearly the power of grace to transform us as well as the way the guru's influence can transform our practice of hatha yoga. The guru, serving as the tangent point between our worldview and the Divine, is a way for the human to experience the Divine in a real and personal way. Instead of God being just another philosophical construct, a relationship with a true guru offers the practitioner a direct experience of the Divine's unconditional love. If we come to such a tangible experience of God's love for us with an open heart, who among us could remain unchanged? If we practice yoga in a way that honors our personal relationship with the Divine, how could we not experience a shift in our practice? And when we glimpse how much we are Loved, how can we dare to keep waging war with ourselves?

Arnaud Desjardins explains his relationship to his guru and the possibility that a genuine guru offers in this way:

> Swamiji brought me back to life on all levels, but being able to rediscover life is something that concerns every human being. For me this image of Lazarus wrapped in graveclothes is a very explicit symbol: you are stiff, you are dead, smothered by the shell of the mind, by fears, false ideas, traumas, illusions, "no's." "No, you don't have the right to live, you don't have the right to love, you don't have the right to breathe, you don't have the right to move, you don't have the right to express yourself, you don't have the right to exist, you have a right to absolutely nothing." And the guru tells you, "Take off your graveclothes, arise, come out of your tomb, come back to life as Lazarus did." Yes . . . opening . . . growth . . . love.[14]

Ending the war with the body is an opening to growth, to love, and to the Divine influence that is ever present and constantly showering its gifts on us.

Obviously everyone who has been at war with the body or who practices yoga will not have a guru. I do and that is my story. Several of the people I interviewed for this project have no established relationship with a spiritual teacher and they have embraced their yoga practice as a practice of peace quite effectively. That is their story. As important as it is to surrender to a guru if that is one's calling, it is equally important to trust where our lives have taken us and to walk the path that is in front of us right now with clarity and certainty. Whether our spiritual life calls us into a relationship with a guru, or into the Roman Catholic Church, or to a campfire in the middle of the forest, or to caring for a sick family member is not so important. What is important in making peace with the body is that we invite the Divine into our hearts, our lives and into our practice of hatha yoga. What is important is that we open our hearts enough to be able to feel the presence of the Divine as It accepts our invitation. What is important is that we begin to cultivate our practice of hatha yoga as a spiritual art.

# CHAPTER EIGHT

# Community: Good Company and the Family of the Heart

*Call it a clan, call it a network, call it a tribe, call it a family.*
*Whatever you call it, whoever you are, you need one.*
                                        —Jane Howard

In the process of making peace with the body and learning to practice yoga from the inside out, we find ourselves in need of sanctuary. Sanctuary is the "shelter from the storm," or the bolstering and support we receive from the community of people with whom we practice.

In the first of Patanjali's *Yoga Sutras,* he says, "Now let us come together to study yoga." Sanskrit scholar Douglas Brooks tells us that this sutra conveys that yoga, in its essence is intended to be a community-oriented pursuit. Just as we join together the body, mind and spirit through the practice of yoga, we can join together as individuals of like mind and heart when we practice. Even in our solitary practice we have the opportunity to align ourselves with the community in subtle ways, feeling connected and supported even in our solitude. Brooks describes the community of practitioners with whom we find sanctuary as the *kula.* Kula is a Sanskrit word he interprets to mean "heart," and more accurately, "the family of the heart."[1]

There are many ways for people to come together. We are born into our family of origin, circumstance dictates our classmates in school, and in many cultures we are brought together by caste or by socio-economic status. The kula, however, is a family in which we *choose* to participate. This family of choice is determined by its members' commitments to sadhana and spiritual awakening, rather than by social obligation or family dictates. The family of the heart might also be called the *sangha* (the term used in Buddhism), or simply *good company* —people who can support us in our process of making peace with our bodies and in our spiritual development. Because cultural messages about our bodies are so strong and the forces that work to destroy our self-image are so pervasive, having others in our life to mirror to us acceptance and encouragement is crucial.

My friend Minnie, quoted earlier, had this to say about community:

> I prefer the company of people who are also deeply committed to their own personal practice and whose influence helps me to remember mine. We all have the power to choose the company we keep. Do we want to be inspired to go beyond our limitations or do we want to be reinforced in believing these false myths?[2]

To expect the Sleeping World to change its values or to expect certain people in our lives to change their orientation to the body and to life in general is unrealistic. Refuge and sanctuary must be sought in a small number of people committed to truth, in the kula. It is with these select few that we share honestly about the work that we are doing to heal from the war on our bodies. We disclose the secrets of our behaviors, our thoughts, and come clean from the pressure of having to appear one way on the surface when something different is happening internally. It is in such sanctuary that we find congruence and authenticity.

Hatha yoga classes have the opportunity to function as reinforcement of the Sleeping World's view or as sanctuary or asylum from the war. Obviously discrimination is called for in this arena—the tone of a community can be one of competition, comparison, vanity and disregard for the body, or one of compassion, empowerment, self-acceptance and encouragement.

Cheryl, a student of Anusara Yoga, speaks about what she has gained by practicing yoga within a community:

> What most definitely what has helped me a lot is that when I walk in here [the yoga studio] I am embraced —and I don't believe that the people in this class see me as a body, they see me as a fellow yogi. And when we applaud each other and when we are so impressed and so inspired by each other, it is really beautiful. And . . . when I am looking around in the larger classes and workshops, when we had twenty-five women in here, we all had different bodies. We all had our own limits and we all had our own challenges and we were all beautiful and we were able to support each other not from a body standpoint but from a loving, compassionate standpoint.
>
> When I walk in here . . . I relax, like, "Here we are." And I don't know if it is unique, but it happens here. And I hope it isn't unique here, because it is one of the main reasons I keep coming back. It isn't just that my body has changed and that my heart has opened more than I ever dreamed before, or that the align-

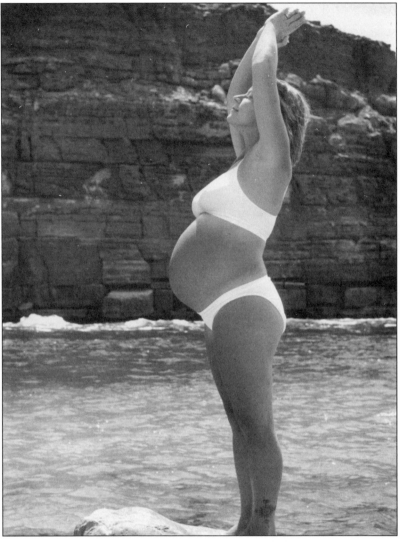

*Urdhva hastasana in tadasana.* Mountain pose.

ment of everything in my life is coming together, but it is also the love and acceptance I feel when I walk in the door.[3]

Like Cheryl did, we can look around in any sizable yoga class and see a myriad of body types practicing yoga with

beauty and grace. We then have a choice to compare ourselves with others or honor ourselves as a unique expression
of the Divine. Our body shape and size or even its age can be
viewed as simply different—no better and no worse than that
of anyone in the room. Allowing ourselves to simply be one
of the group goes a long way toward shifting our perfection-
istic strivings and loosening the grip of our vanity. What if we
didn't have to have a perfect body? What if we simply allowed
ourselves to luxuriate in being average? What if we truly
knew, in every cell of our bodies, that we are lovable exactly
as we are in the moment?

Being part of a group can also help to mirror back to us
our greatness. If we are a part of a group that is committed
to seeing what is possible in us rather than simply what might
be showing up in our personality or body at the moment,
then the group serves a transformational function, not simply a social one.

For many years my main yoga teacher was a person whose
precision and attention to detail was unparalleled. Unfortunately a large amount of his attention was placed on what
was *failing* to happen in my poses rather than on what was
going well. After five years of study with this teacher I didn't
feel like I had any real aptitude for the practice of hatha
yoga. I knew clearly what was wrong with me personally, and
with my practice, but I knew very little about what my
strengths were. Interestingly enough, this teaching style
often created a cold learning environment, with little warmth
generated among the community of practitioners.

Years later I began working with a different teacher who
focused on how to improve on the positive in the asana practice, and on assisting students to open to transformational

possibilities through their yoga practices. I noticed that this openhearted teaching style created an affirming community, or kula, in which I found sanctuary and healing. Being with people who were joining together to celebrate each other's strengths created a generosity within the group that helped to balance the scales of my own self-perception. Positive feedback messages were now added to my "data bank" which had been storing mostly negative impressions of myself. My self-image began to change and my yoga practice at home began showing me the same greatness my fellow students were helping me to see in class.

As a yoga teacher, my teaching style can help to create a supportive community depending on what I emphasize in my classes. It is easy for me to see what is strong and healthy in each of my students. It is equally easy to assess what is scared and underdeveloped in my students. I have a choice to either build on what is positive or to magnify what is negative. By focusing on what is positive I believe we can align ourselves with the practice of making peace, by allowing our weaknesses to be transcended by our strengths. I have the same choices to make when I teach myself in my personal practice. I can chose to focus on my beauty or on my flaws and shortcomings, on love or on neurosis. Albert Einstein's famous words, "You cannot solve a problem at the level of consciousness that it was created," express this spiritual precept succinctly. He was speaking about nuclear war. We are speaking about the war on the body. Both are destructive in their own ways.

Being in a community of practitioners isn't always easy. When we have been in the war zone with our bodies for a long time, we often have the negative thoughts and painful

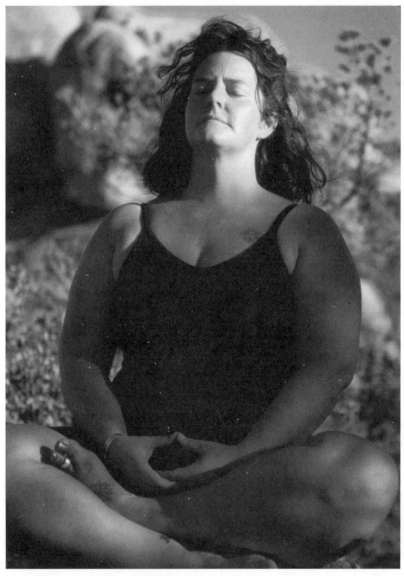

*Arsha padmasana.* Half lotus pose.

feelings that accompany such brutality. Sometimes we are so wounded from our histories that we are unable to see our community clearly. Often being with other people will high-light our tendency to judge ourselves and to compare ourselves with others. Even in the most affirming company it is easy to feel ugly, fat, not good enough and alone.

What hatha yoga can give us, however, are the tools to manage our separative mind games. In the same way that we learn to observe the sensations in our muscles when we perform different asanas, we can notice what is happening with our tendency to compare and to feel inferior. We learn to watch ourselves in community settings, away from the safety of our own solitude. We are indirectly reminded to return to self-observation repeatedly. We practice honoring whatever is arising. We practice holding a compassionate regard for ourselves in the process of unraveling our fears. We can choose to see what is arising as a process of purification, rather than as a flaw in our practice or in ourselves. We can champion ourselves and our efforts, rather than criticizing our practice by being judgmental and harsh.

We might see that the tone of a group practice isn't competitive; rather it is we who are comparing and competing. We may find that even if our friend is dealing with her own war with the body, she may still think our body (with all of our perceived imperfections) is beautiful and inspiring. We may realize that the most "advanced" student in the group is simply another yogi, perfectly imperfect and dealing with his or her own challenges that have nothing to do with our insecurities or with our practice.

As the projections about our community diminish, our expectations of the community will become more realistic. We will be better able to accept people as they are. Our willingness and ability to be nourished by the friendship and support of the kula will increase. We will also be able to serve others, offering back the gifts of the heart that we have so freely been given. We will be able to discern which groups assist us in our growth and which groups are no longer beneficial. We will develop the ability to discriminate what serves our work and what doesn't and we will know what is the best way for us to participate in the kula.

For me, the support of the fellow devotees of my spiritual teacher has been as important in allowing my body image to be transformed as the group of people with whom I practice hatha yoga. Both groups are truly the kula for me, nourishing me and feeding me.

Few of the women in my spiritual community wear makeup or have trendy hairdos. Many are rounder and softer in their physique than the average person I am involved with in fitness or yoga circles. These sangha women are vital and alive, healthy and beautiful, yet in a different way than I have been accustomed to appreciate. When I first began my association with these women I was in the process of severing my ties with the fitness world and ending my addictive relationship with exercise. The fact that I was becoming a part of a community that didn't value body-oriented pursuits and was interested in something deeper than my appearance provided true sanctuary for me. I gained several pounds as my body returned to a more natural relationship with food and exercise, which was simultaneously terrifying, exciting and necessary. One of my sangha sisters continually helped me to feel acceptance about the physical changes I was experiencing, reminding me that as a woman, it was perfectly natural to carry some fat on my hips and around my waist. Many times at the ashram I have heard women sincerely compliment each other when one of them has gained necessary weight. To me this is the power of good company—to lift in-

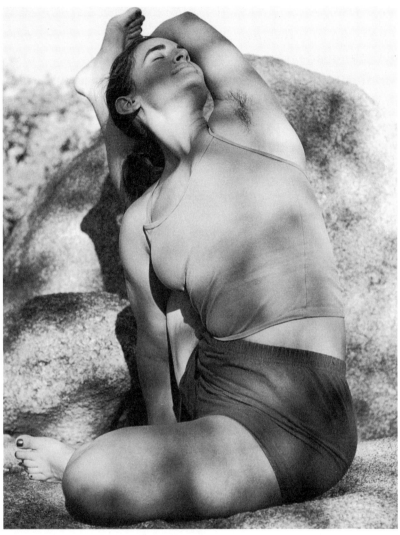

*Surya yantrasana.* Sun dial pose.

dividuals up higher than where they could be on their own. Literally the group subsumes aspects of the individual that are no longer serving that individual's purpose allowing for a greater level of transformation than is possible in isolation.

Tantra can be defined as "looming together or a weaving together." *Tan-* means "to stretch" or "to expand," while *-tra* means "to integrate." This definition of tantra can be used as a metaphor for discussing spiritual community. Each member of the kula might be seen as a thread, that when woven together becomes a tapestry. Thread alone has very little function. It can even be lost or broken quite easily. The value of thread is found in its functioning together with other threads. Thread can be used to mend and it can be used to attach things together. When thread is woven into cloth, the cloth becomes infinitely more useful than a handful of single threads. It is the same for us within a sangha or community— we have the opportunity to be woven into a beautiful cloth. As we bring our individual expression and skills to the group, the group becomes stronger and more functional for service. We, in turn, have function, purpose, strength and stability when bonded in such a way. This bonding creates a continuity of support even when we are not physically surrounded by the ones with whom we practice. This support becomes an internal sanctuary that backs us up and gives us strength to live in the world with the values of a spiritual practitioner.[4]

# Epilogue

*Practice transforms us. We need to eat less, because we assimilate more and more and therefore there is a loss of unnecessary weight. We become more beautiful, our faces change and our walk gains in elasticity. Our way of standing is steady and poised, our legs are firmer, and our toes and feet spread out, giving us more stability. Our chests expand, the muscles of the abdomen start to work, the head is lighter on the neck (like the corolla of a flower on its stem moving easily with flexibility while the wind blows). To watch these enchanting changes is amazing. A different life begins and the body expresses a happiness never felt before. These are not just words; it actually happens.*
—Vanda Scaravelli, *Awakening the Spine*

This book and any other book about spiritual practice can only point the way toward the path. Books can inspire, validate, and perhaps even transmit something essential about the work. But reading about transformation is not the same as being transformed. We must practice. We must do our best in every moment to align ourselves with our intention to make peace and to keep practicing in spite of internal and external obstacles.

Hatha yoga implies the union of opposites. *Ha*—the sun—and *tha*—the moon. I assume this means the opposites within myself as well as the larger opposing forces of the cosmos. We are looking to marry the opposites, to deepen our experience of what the opposites hold or to "live in the tension of opposites," as Carl Jung often taught.[1] For many people yoga is about working hard. For others, yoga is for stress reduction and relaxation only. For some, yoga is for the body. For others, yoga is for the mind. Or perhaps yoga is for the spirit. "Yoga is for moving beyond the body," they say. "Yoga is for moving deeply into the body," others counter, . . . "The body is our temple" . . . "The body is a bag of shit and pus and mucus" . . . "Yoga is for creating flexibility" . . . "Yoga is for developing strength." I think yoga is all of it and more. I think we are best to refrain from rigid definitions or from attempting to nail down this art of yoga too specifically.

Hatha can also mean "to force" or "to strike" or "to resist." In this spirit, hatha can be translated to mean, "to resist habits," to "use force to abstain from what is habitual or conditioned."[2] In making peace with the body, we not only resist the habits of our conditioned mind as it relates to our bodies and our self-perception, but we resist narrowly defining a process that is essentially mysterious. By leaving certain questions unanswered and certain paradoxes unresolved we create room for the magic of the Divine to influence and transform us. We focus our energy on practice and the outcome is left to the will of God. This is surrendered sadhana.

This book has many concepts, suggestions and opinions. Hopefully some of what is offered here will prove to be useful to readers. Using yoga to make peace with the body asks us for an attitude of openness and experimentation as we do our best to follow in the footsteps of so many great sages and saints. Some days the practice of peace will look soft and other days the practice will call for steadfast determination and certain fierceness. We need to know that our relationship to yoga and to ourselves, with yoga as our medium for self-exploration and self-expression, will change. What we can do is to keep going in a context that is fluid and dynamic, with as much love as we can muster.

One of my yoga students also studies dance. She told me a story about attending a workshop with a strict teacher, who was a master of a specific form of Japanese dance. When he was asked questions about the necessity of practice, he replied, "Once you have mastery, it is then that you can truly practice. Even when mastery is attained you must keep going. In fact, all you ever really have is 'keep going'."

I find this story infinitely encouraging. All we may have is keep going. I wonder if we ever really end this process of bringing peace to our bodies through the practice of hatha yoga? I wonder if we would ever really want to stop giving ourselves the gift of this loving attention? What I have been presenting in this book is a process and not a destination. It is a relationship, not a prescription. And like any relationship it will have good days and bad days. Our trust in the relationship may waver. Our trustworthiness will be questionable at times. Our fears will most definitely surface. We will have highs and lows. Our commitment will be challenged. We will want to quit. We may throw in the towel repeatedly. But we must keep going once we decide to bring peace to our bodies and to our practice of hatha yoga.

On the days where we forget to practice entirely we just keep going. On the days where we experience complete freedom from the bondage of self, we keep going. In the midst of our recoil, keep going. In weight loss, keep going. In weight gain, keep going. On easy days, keep going. On difficult days, keep going. When we don't want to anymore, keep going. When we can't imagine any other way, keep going. When we hate God, keep going. When we love God, keep going. Perhaps all we really have is keep going.

*May God bless you as you keep going.*

# *Endnotes*

## CHAPTER ONE: MAKING WAR AND MAKING PEACE

1. *Hohm Sahaj Mandir Study Manual.* Prescott, Arizona: Hohm Press, 1996, p. 609.

## CHAPTER TWO: AWAKENING FROM THE DREAM OF THE SLEEPING WORLD

1. *Hohm Sahaj Mandir Study Manual.* Prescott, Arizona: Hohm Press, 1996, p. 29.

2. *Divine Slave Gita.* "Darshan July 11, 1982." Vol. 2, no. 5, Sept/Oct 1982, pp. 29–30.

3. http://www.emory.edu

4. http://www.healthywithin.com

5. New York Times. "The Tyranny of Skinny, Fashion's Insider Secret." Sunday, March 31, 2002, section 9, p.1.

6. http://www.emory.edu

7. http://www.healthywithin.com

8. http://www.healthywithin.com

9. http://www.emory.edu

10. http://www.healthywithin.com

11. www.healthywithin.com

12. Berman, Marcie. "Yoga and Eating Disorders." *Yoga World,* no. 15, Oct.–Dec. 2000, pp. 8–9.

13. http://www.bksiyengar.com

14. Ji, Minnie. Personal interview, transcripts on file.

## CHAPTER THREE: KAYA SADHANA

1. *Hohm Sahaj Mandir Study Manual.* Prescott, Arizona: Hohm Press, 1996, pp. 140–141

2. Keller, Doug. *Anusara Yoga: Hatha Yoga in the Anusara Style.* South Riding, Virginia: Self-Published, 2001, p. 14.

3. Friend, John. Personal interview, transcripts on file.

4. Martin, Chia. Journal excerpt, transcript on file.

5. Ramano, Ria. "Yoga: A Path of Optimization," *Counselor Magazine,* October 2001, p. 48.

## CHAPTER FOUR: PAYING ATTENTION

1. *Hohm Sahaj Mandir Study Manual.* Prescott, Arizona: Hohm Press, 1996, p. 349.

2. Friend, John. *Anusara Yoga Teacher Training Manual.* Shenandoah, Texas: Anusara Press, 1999, p. 29.

3. Feuerstein, Georg. *The Yoga Sutra of Patanjali: A New Translation and Commentary.* Rochester, Vermont: Inner Traditions International, 1979.

## CHAPTER FIVE: OPENING THE HEART: UNCOVERING AND EXPRESSING OUR TRUE NATURE

1. *Hohm Sahaj Mandir Study Manual.* Prescott, Arizona: Hohm Press, 1996, p. 20.

2. Incao, Sylvan. "One Month in France with the Spiritual Master, July 2001." *Tawagoto,* vol. 14, no.4, Fall 2001, p. 23.

3. Chögyam Trungpa Rinpoche. *Shambhala: The Sacred Path of the Warrior.* New York: Bantam, 1987, p. 31.

4. Brooks, Douglas. Lecture notes, on file.

5. Brooks, Douglas. Lecture notes, on file.

6. Ryan, Regina Sara. *Praying Dangerously: Radical Reliance on God.* Prescott, Arizona: Hohm Press, 2001, pp. 78–79.

7. Brooks, Douglas. Lecture notes, on file.

8. Brooks, Douglas. Lecture notes, on file.

9. Ryan, pp. 78–79.

## CHAPTER SIX: ACCEPTING "WHAT IS"

1. Surtemps and Dia. "Arnaud Desjardins at Ferme De Jutreau." *Tawagoto,* vol. 14, no.4, Fall 2001, p. 58.

2. Desjardins, Arnaud. *The Jump Into Life: Moving Beyond Fear.* Prescott, Arizona: Hohm Press, 1994, p. 136.

3. Desjardins, p. 138.

4. Friend, John. *Anusara Yoga Teacher Training Manual.* Shenandoah, Texas: Anusara Press, 1999, p. 20.

5. Dworkis, Sam (2001). www.extensionyoga.com

6. Klostermaier, Klaus K. *A Concise Encyclopedia of Hinduism.* Oxford: One World, 1998, p. 141.

7. Auletta, Deborah. Personal interview, on file.

8. Auletta, Deborah. Personal interview, on file.

9. Lozowick, Lee. Personal interview, on file.

10. Friend, John. Personal interview, on file.

11. Friend, John. Personal interview, on file.

## CHAPTER SEVEN: HATHA YOGA AS A SPIRITUAL ART

1. Lozowick, Lee. Personal correspondence, on file.

2. Feuerstein, Trisha Lamb. Personal correspondence, on file.

3. Feuerstein, Georg. *Tantra: The Path of Ecstasy.* Boston, Massachusetts: Shambhala Publications, 1998, p. 93.

4. Ibid, p.18.

5. Freud, Sigmund. *Civilization and Its Discontents.* New York, New York: W.W. Norton and Company, 1961, pp. 53–63.

6. Gold, E.J. *The Great Adventure.* Nevada City, California: Gateway Books and Tapes, 2001, pp. 6–7.

7. *Hohm Sahaj Mandir Study Manual.* Prescott, Arizona: Hohm Press, 1996, p. 574.

8. Ibid.

9. Feuerstein, Georg. p. 88.

10. Feuerstein, Georg. p. 89, and *Hohm Sahaj Mandir* p. 26.

11. Feuerstein, Georg. p. 93.

12. Feuerstein, Georg, p. 18.

13. Friend, John. Personal interview, transcripts on file.

14. Desjardins, Arnaud. *The Jump Into Life: Moving Beyond Fear.* Prescott, Arizona: Hohm Press, 1994, p. 148.

## CHAPTER EIGHT: COMMUNITY

1. Brooks, Douglas. Lecture notes, on file.

2. Ji, Minnie. Personal interview, transcripts on file.

3. Walters, Cheryl. Personal interview, transcripts on file.

4. Brooks, Douglas. Lecture notes, on file.

## EPILOGUE: KEEP GOING

1. *The Basic Writings of C.G. Jung.* (Ed.) Violet Staub de Lasto. New York: Random House, 1993, p. 222.

2. Brooks, Douglas. Lecture notes, on file.

# Recommended Reading

Caplan, Mariana. *Do You Need A Guru?* London: Thorsons, 2002.

Chodron, Pema. *When Things Fall Apart: Heart Advice for Difficult Times.* Boston: Shambhala, 1997.

Cope, Stephen. *Yoga and The Quest for the True Self.* New York: Bantam, 1999.

Desjardins, Arnaud. *The Jump Into Life: Moving Beyond Fear.* Prescott, Arizona: Hohm Press.

Feuerstein, Georg. Tantra: *The Path of Ecstasy.* Boston: Shambhala, 1998.

Friend, John. *Anusara Yoga Teacher Training Manual.* Shenandoah, Texas: Anusara Press, 1999.

Gannon, Sharon and Life, David. *Jivamukti Yoga: Practices for Liberating Body and Soul.* New York: Ballantine Books, 2002.

Gold, E.J. *The Great Adventure.* Nevada City, California: Gateways Books and Tapes, 2001.

Incao, Sylvan. *Zen Trash: Irreverent and Sacred Teaching Stories of Lee Lozowick*. Prescott, Arizona, 2002.

Iyengar, B.K.S. *Light on Pranayama*. New York: Crossroad Publishing, 1994.

Iyengar, B.K.S. *TheTree of Yoga*. Boston: Shambhala, 2002.

Keller, Doug. *Anusara Yoga: Hatha Yoga in the Anusara Style*. South Riding, Virginia: Self-Published, 2001.

Lasater, Judith. *Relax and Renew: Restful Yoga for Stressful Times*. Berkeley, California: Rodmell Press, 1995.

Mehta, Silva. *Yoga The Iyengar Way: The New Definitive Illustrated Guide*. New York: Alfred A. Knopf, 1996.

Myers, Esther. *Yoga and You: Energizing and Relaxing Yoga for New and Experienced Students*. Boston: Shambhala, 1997.

Ryan, Regina Sara. *Praying Dangerously: Radical Reliance on God*. Prescott, Arizona: Hohm Press, 2001.

Scaravelli, Vanda. *Awakening the Spine: The Stress-free New Yoga that Works with the Body to Restore Health, Vitality and Energy*. New York: Harper Collins Publishers, 1991.

Shiffman, Erich. *Yoga: The Spirit and Practice of Moving Into Stillness*. New York: Pocket Books, 1996.

Stiles, Mukunda. *Yoga Sutras of Patanjali*. Boston: Weiser Books, 2002.

Trungpa Rinpoche, Chögyam. *Crazy Wisdom*. Boston: Shambhala, 1991.

# *Index*

## THE YOGA TRADITION
*History, Literature, Philosophy and Practice*
by Georg Feuerstein, Ph.D.
Foreword by Ken Wilber

A complete overview of the great Yogic traditions of: Raja-Yoga, Hatha-Yoga, Jnana-Yoga, Bhakti-Yoga, Karma-Yoga, Tantra-Yoga, Kundalini-Yoga, Mantra-Yoga and many other lesser known forms. Includes translations of over twenty famous Yoga treatises, like the *Yoga-Sutra of Patanjali,* and a first-time translation of the *Goraksha Paddhati,* an ancient Hatha Yoga text. Covers all aspects of Hindu, Buddhist, Jaina and Sikh Yoga. A necessary resource for all students and scholars of Yoga.

Paper, 550 pages, more than 200 illustrations, $29.95
ISBN: 1-8990772-18-6

## HALFWAY UP THE MOUNTAIN
*The Error of Premature Claims to Enlightenment*
by Mariana Caplan

Author and anthropologist Mariana Caplan plunges into the complex domain of contemporary spirituality where she boldly faces the grave distortions and fraudulent claims to power that characterize the spiritual path in our times. Dozens of first-hand interviews with students, respected teachers and masters, together with broad research are synthesized into a treatment of the modern spiritual scene to assist readers in avoiding the pitfalls of this precarious path. With original contributions from: Charles Tart, Ph.D., Andrew Cohen, Robert Svoboda, Joan Halifax,, Georg Feuerstein, Lee Lozowick, Jokshu Kwong Roshi, Dr. Reginald Ray, Llewellyn Vaughn-Lee, and others.

Paper; 600 pages; $21.95
ISBN: 934252-91-2

## TO TOUCH IS TO LIVE
*The Need for Genuine Affection in an Impersonal World*
by Mariana Caplan, Ph.D.
Foreword by Ashley Montagu

The vastly impersonal nature of contemporary culture, supported by massive child abuse and neglect, and reinforced by growing techno-fascination are robbing us of our humanity. The author takes issue with the trends of the day that are mostly overlooked as being "progressive" or harmless, showing how these trends are actually undermining genuine affection and love. This uncompromising and inspiring work offers positive solutions for countering the effects of the growing depersonalization of our times.

*"To all of us with bodies, in an increasingly disembodied world, this book comes as a passionate reminder that: Touch is essential to health and happiness."*

**—Joanna Macy,**
author of *World as Lover, World as Self*

*"Mariana discusses virtually every significant human need and behavior in a language that abjures all technical terms, and speaks plainly and simply, both to the heart and the mind's consent. This is a considerable achievement."*

**—Ashley Montagu,**
author of *Touching, The Human Significance of the Skin*

Paper, 270 pages, $19.95
ISBN: 1-890772-24-0

## AS IT IS
*A Year on the Road with a Tantric Teacher*
by M. Young

A first-hand account of a one-year journey around the world in the company of *tantric* teacher Lee Lozowick. This book catalogues the trials and wonders of day-to-day interactions between a teacher and his students, and presents a broad range of his teachings given in seminars from San Francisco, California to Rishikesh, India. *As It Is* considers the core principles of *tantra*, including non-duality, compassion (the Bodhisattva ideal), service to others, and transformation within daily life. Written as a narrative, this captivating book will appeal to practitioners of *any* spiritual path. Readers interested in a life of clarity, genuine creativity, wisdom and harmony will find this an invaluable resource.

Paper, 840 pages, 24 b&w photos, $29.95
ISBN: 0-934252-99-8


## THE JUMP INTO LIFE
*Moving Beyond Fear*
by Arnaud Desjardins
Foreword by Richard Moss, M.D.

"Say Yes to life," the author continually invites in this welcome guidebook to the spiritual path. For anyone who has ever felt oppressed by the life-negative seriousness of religion, this book is a timely antidote. In language that translates the complex to the obvious, Desjardins applies his simple teaching of happiness and gratitude to a broad range of weighty topics, including sexuality and intimate relationships, structuring an "inner life," the relief of suffering, and overcoming fear.

Paper, 278 pages, $12.95
ISBN: 0-934252-42-4

## THE ALCHEMY OF TRANSFORMATION

by Lee Lozowick
Foreword by Claudio Naranjo, M.D.

A concise and straightforward overview of the principles of spiritual life as developed and taught by Lee Lozowick for the past twenty years. Subjects of use to seekers and serious students of any spiritual tradition include: A radical, elegant and irreverent approach to the possibility of change from ego-centeredness to God-centeredness—the ultimate human transformation.

Paper, 192 pages, $14.95
ISBN: 0-934252-62-9

## WOMEN CALLED TO THE PATH OF RUMI
### *The Way of the Whirling Dervish*
by Shakina Reinhertz

This book shares the experience of Turning practice by women of the Mevlevi Order of Whirling Dervishes. The beauty and mystery of the Whirling Dervishes have captured the mythic imagination of the Western world for centuries. Rumi, the great Sufi saint of 13th-century Turkey, taught both male and female students this whirling dance, but in the centuries after his death women were excluded from participation. Not until the late 1970s, when Shaikh Suleyman Dede brought the turn ritual to America, was this practice again opened to women. The heart of the book is the personal experience of contemporary women interviews over two dozen American initiates (from adolescents to wise elders), many of whom have practiced on this path for twenty years or more.

*"I love the wisdom and fire of this book. It's full of the light of longing and people trying to experience the mystery of that truth."*

**—Coleman Barks**,
translator of Rumi's poetry.

Paper, 300 pages; 200 b&w photos and illustrations; $23.95
ISBN: 1-890772-04-6

## THE WOMAN AWAKE
*Feminine Wisdom for Spiritual Life*
by Regina Sara Ryan

Through the stories and insights of great women whom the author has met or been guided by in her own journey, this book highlights many faces of the Divine Feminine: the silence, the solitude, the service, the power, the compassion, the art, the darkness, the sexuality. Read about: the Sufi poetess Rabia (8th century) and contemporary Sufi master Irina Tweedie; Hildegard of Bingen, author Kathryn Hulme (*The Nun's Story*), German healer and mystic Dina Rees, and others. Includes personal interviews with contemplative Christian monk Mother Tessa Bielecki; artist Meinrad Craighead and Zen teacher and anthropologist Joan Halifax.

Paper; 20 photos; 518 pages; $19.95
ISBN: 0-934252-79-3

## PRAYING DANGEROUSLY
*Radical Reliance on God*
by Regina Sara Ryan

*Praying Dangerously* re-enlivens an age-old tradition of prayer as an expression of radical reliance on God, or non-compromising surrender to Life *as it is.* This approach expands the possibilities of prayer, elevating it beyond ordinary pleas for help, comfort, security and prosperity. *Praying Dangerously* invites a renewal of the inner life, by increasing one's desire to burn away superficial, safe notions of God, holiness, satisfaction and peace.

*"A brave book for brave people . . ."*
—**David Steindl-Rast,** O.S.B.,
author *Gratefulness, the Heart of Prayer*

*". . . wise, fierce, challenging . . ."*
—**Andrew Harvey,**
author *The Essential Mystics*

Paper, 240 pages, $14.95
ISBN: 1-8990772-06-2

**Visit our website at www.hohmpress.com**

## JOURNEY
### From Political Activism to the Work
by Janet Rose

This book recounts the story of a spiritual journey that led the author from a life of political and social activism to a life of spiritual transformation. Having worked as a newspaper reporter, a manager of a food cooperative, a coordinator of a rural health service and a VISTA volunteer, Janet Rose thought her next step was to build her practice as a psychotherapist in a large southeastern city. In the summer of 1986, however, almost overnight her life took a radical turn. Following inner mystical guidance, she turned west, to the mountains of Colorado, to "find God more deeply." In her quest for genuine wisdom, compassion and service, she left behind the vestiges of her previous life to pursue a path of renunciation and to apprentice herself to a spiritual teacher. How that choice was made, what that commitment entailed, and how it has changed every aspect of her life is what this book is about.

Paper, 384 pages, $19.95
ISBN: 1-890772-04-6

## 10 ESSENTIAL FOODS
by Lalitha Thomas

Carrots, broccoli, almonds, grapefruit and six other miracle foods will enhance your health when used regularly and wisely. Lalitha gives in-depth nutritional information plus flamboyant and good-humored stories about these foods, based on her years of health and nutrition counseling. Each chapter contains easy and delicious recipes, tips for feeding kids and helpful hints for managing your food dollar. A bonus section supports the use of 10 Essential Snacks.

Paper, 300 pages, $16.95
ISBN: 0-934252-74-2

**INTUITIVE EATING**
*EveryBody's Guide to Vibrant Health and Lifelong Vitality Through Food*
by Humbart "Smokey" Santillo, N.D.

The natural voice of the body has been drowned out by the shouts of addictions, over-consumption, and devitalized and preserved foods. Millions battle the scale daily, experimenting with diets and nutritional programs, only to find their victories short-lived at best, confusing and demoralizing at worst. Intuitive Eating offers an alternative a tested method for: • strengthening the immune system • natural weight loss • increasing energy • making the transition from a degenerative diet to a regenerative diet • slowing the aging process.

Paper, 450 pages, $16.95
ISBN: 0-934252-27-0

Visit our website at www.hohmpress.com

# HOHM PRESS

Name _____ Phone _____

Address or P.O. Box _____

City _____ State _____ Zip_____

| QTY | TITLE | PRICE | TOTAL |
|-----|-------|-------|-------|
| | The Yoga Tradition | $29.95 | |
| | Halfway Up the Mountain | $21.95 | |
| | To Touch is to Live | $19.95 | |
| | As It Is | $29.95 | |
| | The Jump Into Life | $12.95 | |
| | The Alchemy of Transformation | $14.95 | |
| | Women Called to the Path of Rumi | $23.95 | |
| | The Woman Awake | $19.95 | |
| | Praying Dangerously | $14.95 | |
| | Journey | $19.95 | |
| | 10 Essential Foods | $16.95 | |
| | Intuitive Eating | $16.95 | |
| | Yoga From the Inside Out | $14.95 | |

**Surface Shipping Charges**

| | | *Subtotal* | |
|---|---|---|---|
| 1st book | $5.00 | | |
| Each additional item | $1.00 | *Shipping* | |

**Method of Shipping**

**TOTAL**

_____ Surface U.S. Mail (Priority)

_____ 2nd-Day Air Mail (Mail +$5.00)

_____ FedEx Ground (Mail +$3.00)

_____ Next-Day Air Mail (Mail +$15.00)

**Visit our website to view our complete catalog!**

**Method of Payment**

_____ Check or M.O.—Payable to Hohm Press

_____ Call 800.381.2700 to place a credit card order

_____ Call 928.717.1779 to fax a credit card order

**www.hohmpress.com**

**Credit Card Information**

Card # _____ Exp. Date _____

By request, Christina Sell leads yoga workshops in North America and Europe. Further information can be found at www.prescottyoga.com or by writing to her

c/o: Hohm Press
   Box 2501, Prescott
   Arizona, 86302, U.S.A.